CRIME LABS

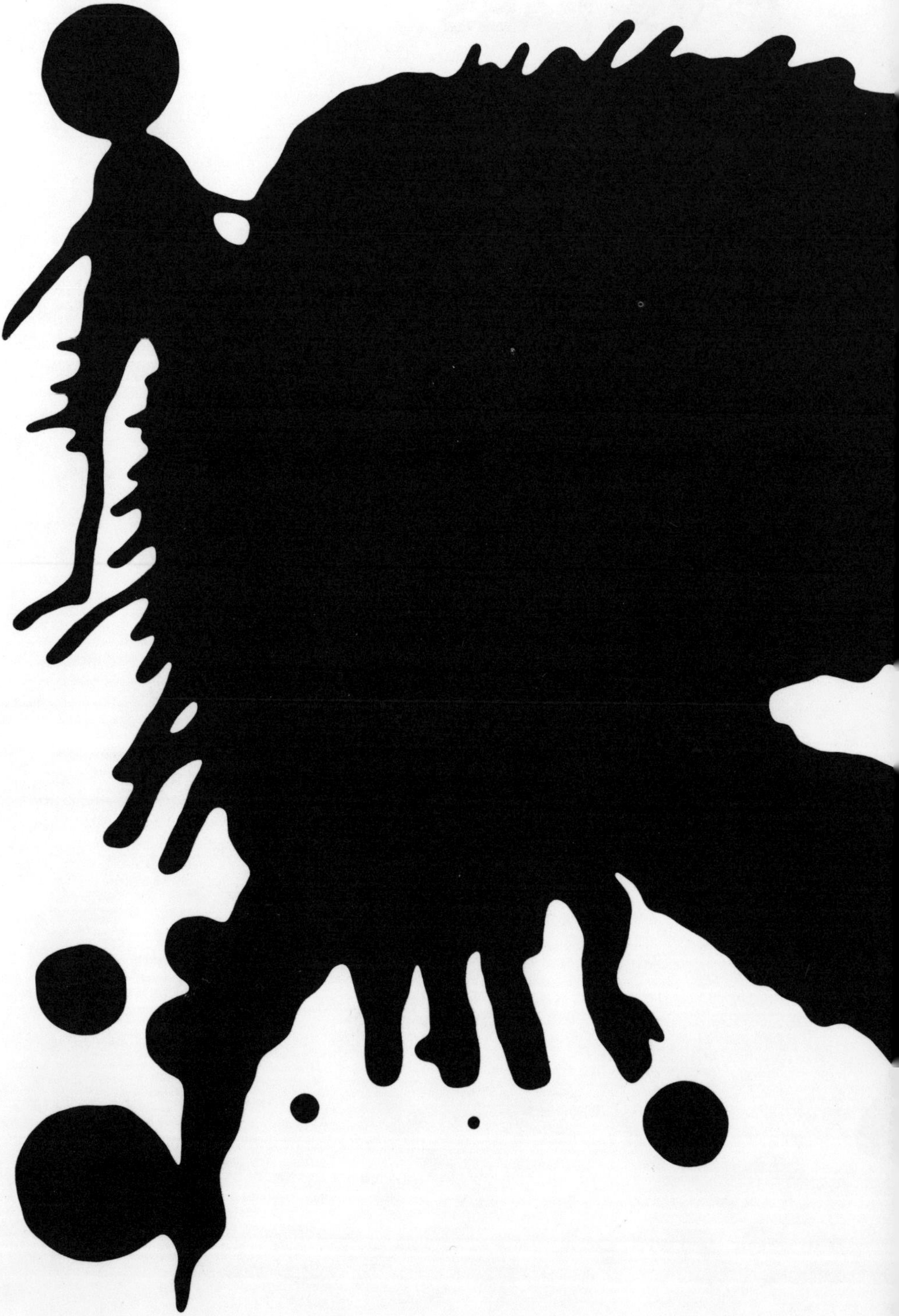

CRIME LABS

THE SCIENCE OF FORENSIC MEDICINE

by John F. Waters

FRANKLIN WATTS
NEW YORK | LONDON | 1979
AN IMPACT BOOK

Photographs courtesy of: *Spring 3100,* N.Y.P.D. magazine: pp. 8, 29, 69; *Law and Order* magazine: pp. 11, 42, (James E. Lubbock) 74; FBI: pp. 21, 24; Erie County Laboratory: pp. 32, 35; *Law Enforcement Communications* magazine, photo by Dr. Lowell Levine, Medical Examiner's Office: p. 49; Unitron Instruments, Inc., a subsidiary of Ehrenreich Photo-Optical Industries, Inc.: p. 60.

Library of Congress Cataloging in Publication Data

Waters, John Frederick, 1930–
Crime labs: the science of forensic medicine.

(An Impact book)
Bibliography: p.
Includes index.
SUMMARY: Discusses the role of forensic medicine in the solution of crimes and describes the jobs of various experts involved in this process.
1. Crime laboratories—Juvenile literature. 2. Criminal investigation—Juvenile literature. 3. Forensic pathology—Juvenile literature. [1. Crime laboratories. 2. Criminal investigation. 3. Forensic pathology] I. Title.
HV8073.W38 614'.19 78–23890
ISBN 0–531–02286–2

Printed in the United States of America
6 5 4 3 2 1

CONTENTS

!MPACT BOOKS provide a thorough introduction to contemporary topics.

BIONICS
BIORHYTHM
THE COLONIAL CONQUEST OF ASIA
CRIME AND CAPITAL PUNISHMENT
CRIME LABS
DRIFTING CONTINENTS, SHIFTING SEAS
THE ECONOMIC GROWTH DEBATE
ESP
FAMINE
GENEALOGY
GEOLOGICAL DISASTERS
GUN CONTROL
LEARNING DISABILITIES AND HANDICAPS
NAVIGATION
THE NEW ICE AGE
PRIMARIES AND CONVENTIONS
SEARCH FOR LIFE BEYOND EARTH
SOLAR ENERGY
SPACE TECHNOLOGY SPINOFFS
SUPERCOLD/SUPERHOT
UNDERSTANDING BODY TALK
UNDERSTANDING TODAY'S ECONOMICS
WATER: A SCARCE RESOURCE

CRIME LABS

THE CRIME

When the police stepped through the door of the bedroom, they saw a gruesome scene. One policeman stated that he'd never seen anything like it before, and he had been on the force for almost thirty years. On the floor of the bedroom they found a prominent heart specialist, shot through the head. A gun lay nearby, next to his outstretched right hand. His wife was on the bed. She too had been shot, once in the chest and twice in the head. On a first impression one might have labeled the case as murder and then suicide. It appeared that the doctor had shot his wife and then had turned the gun to his head and taken his own life.

However, there was police work to be done. A medical investigator, Dr. Paul Fisk, arrived to view the crime scene. Teams of men and women began collecting evidence. They took photographs of the entire room and everything in it. They found what they thought were human hairs on the rug and bed. They found smudge marks and blood on the carpet, so they cut out that part of the carpet and took it to their laboratory. When all available evidence was gathered, the bodies were released to the morgue to be examined by a coroner, a physician trained in the examination of deceased victims of crimes.

The police were very interested in the case because they were not sure if it was a murder-suicide, as it appeared, and therefore an open-and-shut case, or if it was a double murder. Insurance companies were very interested because of the high amount of life insurance the dead doctor carried. If, indeed, he was a suicide, then the insurance companies would not have to pay out a half-million dollars to the younger sister of the doctor. There were no children. If it was a double murder, then the insurance companies would have to pay.

Police Detective Frank Rogers, who was forty-five years old with seventeen years as a detective of the city of DePault (population 1,440,000), was assigned to the case. He was to investigate the deaths of Dr. Theodore Morgan, semiretired heart specialist, and his wife Ruth, who was active in many civic affairs throughout DePault. Both were well known in the city, respected and liked, and their deaths made the front page of the *DePault Daily Enterprise.*

Detective Rogers had three immediate suspects who had access to the family and who had possible motives for committing the murders. There was Amanda Hale, the maid, who had been at home and asleep, so she said, at the time of the shootings. There was Dr. Morgan's younger sister, Beatrice. She was married to an unemployed salesman, had five children, and was in financial trouble. She had a motive: the insurance policies. A third immediate suspect was George, the gardener who had occasionally mowed lawns and raked leaves for the Morgans. He had worked for the Morgans for five years before quitting after an argument, about a month before the shootings. George had stated many times that he was going to get even with the Morgans because, he said, they owed him a week's salary.

When Detective Rogers arrived, he found the bedroom fairly neat, with nothing out of place except for a small drawer open on the night table that belonged to Mrs. Morgan. The contents of the drawer—gloves, handkerchiefs, hair nets, stockings—were in disarray, as though someone had been hurriedly searching through them for something. There was no sign of a struggle.

Rogers made notes of what he saw. He still didn't know if he was dealing with a suicide or a double murder. He hesitated to approach any of the suspects until he had a full lab report from the medical examiner. An extensive investigation would not be necessary if it was determined that the doctor had killed himself, so Rogers decided to have the room sealed off, pending the examination. He then went back to the police station to work on another case until he was called by the coroner to be present during the autopsy.

(4)

THE ROLE OF THE DOCTOR

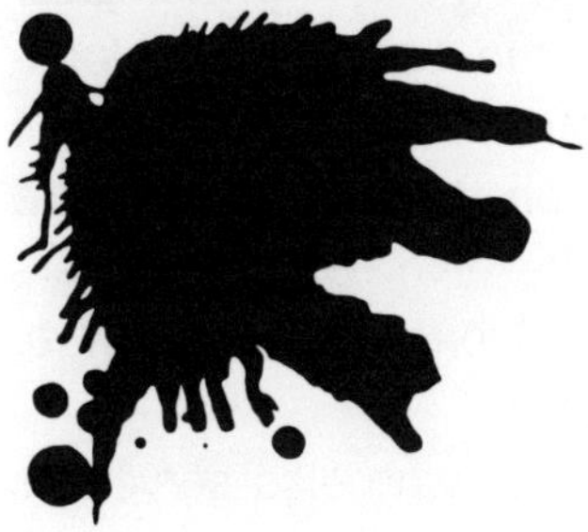

Shortly after the bodies were discovered, the police called in a doctor known as a medical investigator to examine the bodies at the scene. The medical investigator determined that both were indeed dead and that death probably could be attributed to gunshot wounds. An approximate time of death was established, and the medical investigator made notes about the position of the bodies and bloodstains around the room. When he was finished, crime lab personnel went to work, and when they were done, the medical investigator supervised the two police officers who placed the bodies in rubberized bags for delivery to the laboratory of the medical examiner.

Dr. Fearing Schultz, a pathologist who also served as the city coroner, was called in. He waited in the city laboratory to do a complete autopsy as soon as the bodies were delivered. With the help of lab assistants, he examined the outside of the body before he cut open Mrs. Morgan to look for any evidence of other injury or disease. He examined the heart, brain, kidneys, and other organs. He also took blood samples and urine samples and examined the stomach contents.

Dr. Schultz then performed an autopsy on Dr. Morgan as he had with Mrs. Morgan. He made a careful study of the gunshot wound to the head. He noted the point of entry of the bullet and examined the wound for any evidence of powder burns. He knew that burns to the skin are evident when a gun is fired at close range. Dr. Morgan was also dissected and his vital organs examined. Samples of his body fluids were taken. After more than three hours of examination, Dr. Schultz formed his opinion of what had happened. He was then ready to make his report to the police, and to Detective Rogers in particular.

Not all doctors work with the results of a crime as much as Dr. Schultz does, of course. Family doctors are occasionally called upon to treat patients with accidentally inflicted knife or gunshot wounds, but such cases are out of the ordinary for most family doctors. (Doctors are required to report such cases to the police.) However, many doctors, especially in the beginning of their careers, are asked to take shifts in the emergency room of a hospital. In the emergency room they may see the results of crime more often. Many people brought to hospital emergency rooms are victims of stabbings or shootings, or people with injuries from hit-and-run traffic accidents.

But, for doctors who choose to work as medical examiners, as Dr. Schultz did, the exposure to crime is almost constant. As a pathologist, Dr. Schultz is a specialist who concentrates on discovering the nature and function of disease. His job is to open the body and examine all internal organs, as he did with the bodies of Dr. Morgan and his wife. During the examination, the pathologist looks for any signs that will indicate what the cause of death might have been. For instance, death might have been caused by disease, accidental injury, or injury deliberately inflicted by another human being.

If a pathologist cannot find any cause of death—even after examination of the kidneys, brain, liver, heart, and the body fluids—then a toxicologist may be called in. The toxicologist is not a medical doctor, but a scientist familiar with the chemical makeup of poisons and their effects on the human body.

When a victim of a suspected poisoning is brought in, the toxicologist tries to isolate the poison from the body tissue. Once the poison is extracted, the next step is to identify the substance. Following identification, the toxicologist attempts to estimate how much poison is in the body and tries to determine whether this amount would be considered a lethal dose.

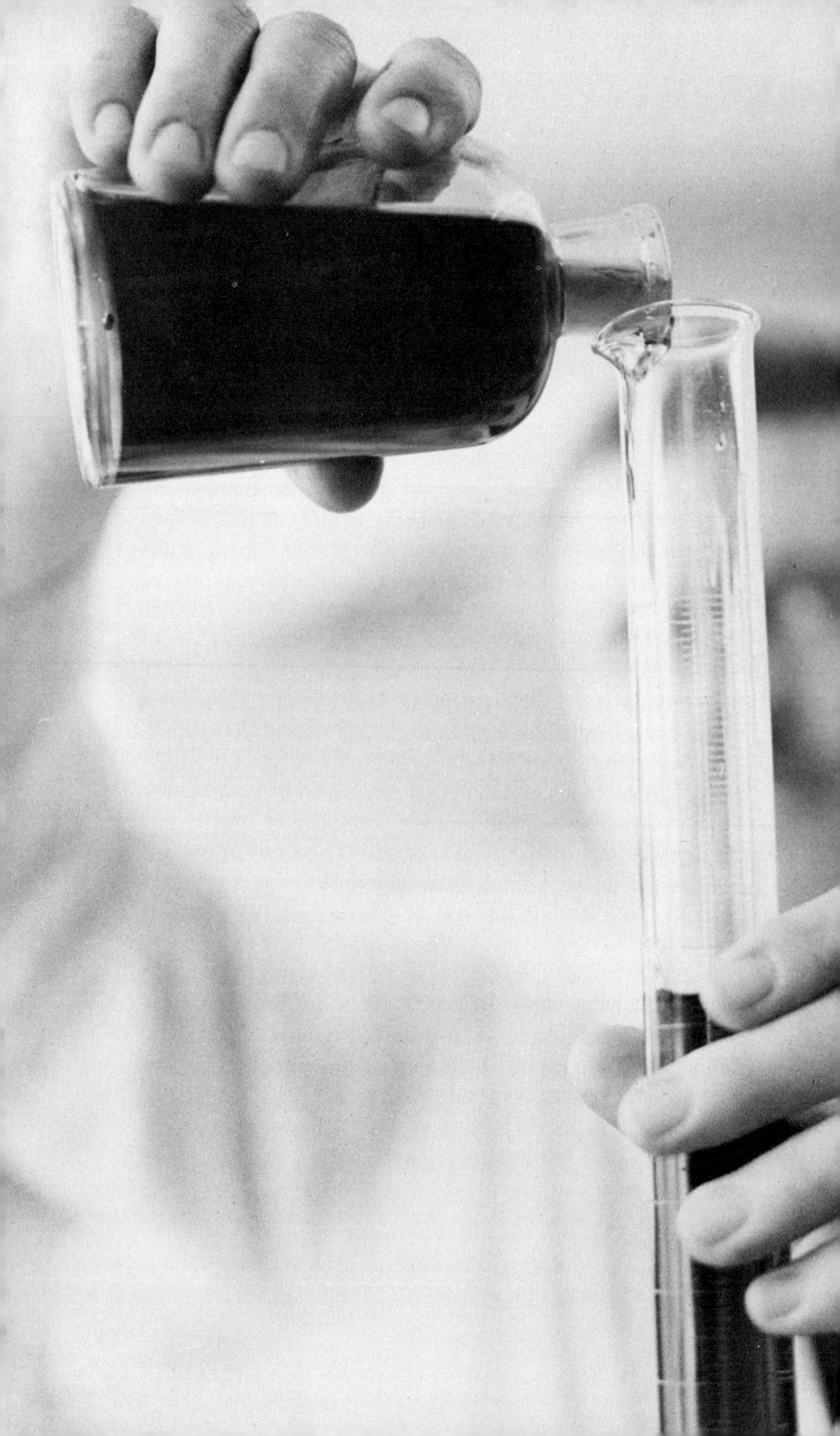

Going back to the case of Dr. Morgan and his wife: no poisons were found in either body. They did not die of natural causes. It was established that Mrs. Morgan died of gunshots, fired from some distance. Dr. Morgan died as a result of a gunshot to the head. Because no traces of powder burns were found at the wound, Dr. Schultz determined that the shot which killed Dr. Morgan was also fired from a distance. In addition to checking for powder burns, Dr. Schultz also examined the angle of the wound, which showed the way the bullet entered the head. This, too, indicated that Dr. Morgan had not shot himself, because the angle at which the bullet entered the skull was not what it would have been if he had fired the gun himself. Dr. Schultz decided that the gunshot was inflicted by a third party.

Now Detective Rogers had a case to work on. Someone else had definitely been in the room and fired the gun. But who? Frank Rogers turned to the medical investigator, Dr. Fisk, for help.

When Dr. Fisk had arrived on the scene of the Morgan murders, he was careful to bring nothing into the bedroom except his medical bag. This was to avoid bringing any foreign matter, such as the ash from a lighted cigarette, into the room, where it might be mistakenly gathered as evidence to be processed at the crime laboratory. Dr. Fisk took out his pencil and notebook and made notes describing how the bodies were arranged, what clothing was worn, and how the clothing was arranged. He felt the

TOXICOLOGY IS AN
ESSENTIAL BRANCH OF
FORENSIC MEDICINE.

foreheads of both victims to check their body temperature and then estimated that the time of death had been 7:30 A.M. When he was finished determining time of death, he allowed the crime laboratory people to come into the room and begin their work.

Determining time of death is one of the medical investigator's most important functions. In the case of the double murder of the Morgans, the time of death ruled out two of the suspects immediately—Beatrice, the younger sister, and George, the fired gardener. Both, it was later learned, had ironclad excuses and were far from the scene of the crime when the two were shot. That left only the maid, who claimed to have been asleep down the hall. Rogers did not consider her as a logical suspect, however, since she had been with the Morgans for years and was considered to be a part of the family.

Once the crime lab people were finished collecting evidence, the medical investigator returned and took charge of removing the bodies to the mortuary for examination. At the mortuary, crime lab scientists went over both bodies before Dr. Schultz began his autopsy. Dr. Schultz removed all clothing from the bodies, piece by piece, and wrapped and labeled everything. All loose hairs, fibers, and bits of foreign material were collected, sealed in plastic, and labeled. Scrapings were taken from the lips and skin, as well as from the fingernails, for later examination at the crime lab. Full sets of photographs were taken of both bodies.

A PORTABLE CRIME LAB
IS TAKEN TO THE SCENE.

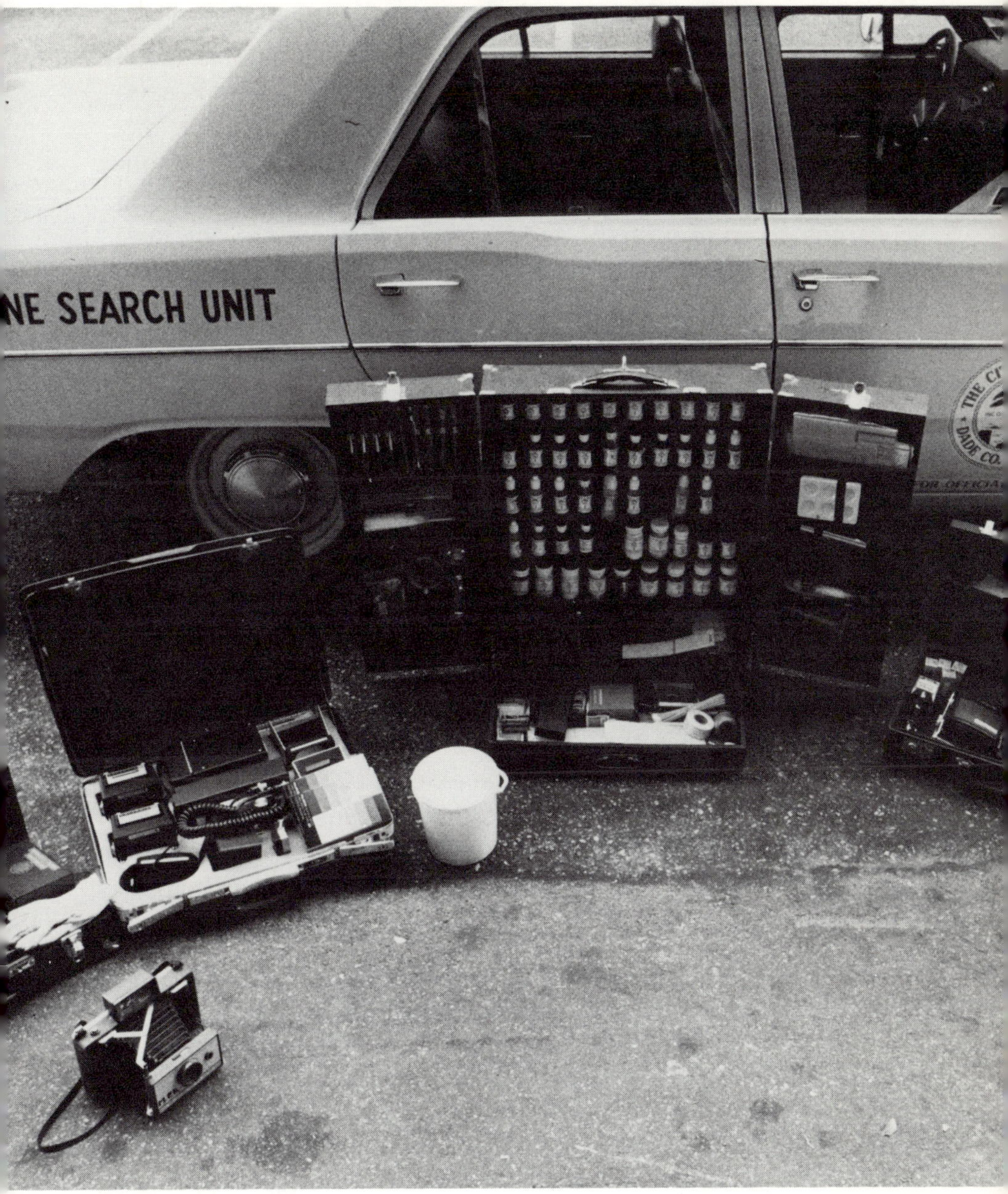
NE SEARCH UNIT

It is important to note that every item of evidence is sealed, wrapped, and identified for a reason. This material is turned over to the police and locked up for safekeeping. In this case, Detective Rogers handled the evidence. No one can see the evidence without proper authority and without signing for it. This practice is called the chain of custody, and is designed to prevent any tampering with the evidence. A courtroom lawyer could have evidence thrown out of court if it was shown that any evidence had been carelessly handled, making tampering possible.

Dr. Schultz removed the vital organs for further examination. In many cases, vital organs are removed for additional study because in court the pathologist may be asked if someone died of natural causes or poisoning before being shot as charged by the district attorney. It is important that the pathologist make a thorough examination and know as much as possible about the deceased. In the Morgan case, a smart lawyer could try to discredit the findings of the pathologist in court in order to raise the possibility that the victims were dead before they were shot. The pathologist must be able to state that there was no question that both victims died of gunshot wounds and nothing else.

When Dr. Schultz was satisfied with his examination, he released the bodies for burial and recorded all his findings on paper, with photographs, and on a tape recording. His records included written reports, photographs, and the tape-recorded observations. All this would be held on file and would be available if the case came to trial. The report was also available to Detective Rogers. If Rogers does find a suspect and gathers enough evidence to warrant an arrest, then the district attorney will hold a hearing. The pathologist is required to attend that hearing. Dr. Schultz will state that the two victims were shot and that their deaths were due to their gunshot wounds. He will also testify that none of the wounds was self-inflicted. If all goes well, the case will then go to trial.

During the trial, the pathologist will be asked to give testimony. He or she will present all the medical evidence available. The pathologist will answer all medical questions about the deceased asked by the prosecutor and by the lawyer defending the suspect. If the doctor has performed well, he or she will be able to answer all questions thoroughly and professionally.

EARLY LEGAL MEDICINE

Today it is common practice for medical doctors to testify in the courtroom because they have knowledge of criminal cases. But is this a new practice, or has it been just in the twentieth century that various medical experts have been asked to give evidence regarding crimes? It may seem new, but actually the earliest application of medicine to criminal investigation took place before the birth of Christ. Members of early tribes tried to determine if a death was by accident, by natural causes, murder, or suicide. This was most important even then, because tribal customs denied funeral rites to suicides since it was thought that anyone who took his or her own life was possessed by the devil. In some primitive African tribes, the hut of the suicide was burned to the ground and the remaining family was ousted from the tribe.

In ancient Rome, soldiers who took their own lives were considered to be deserters. During the tenth century in England, suicide was considered to be a crime, and later the Roman Catholic Church condemned suicide as sinful.

One of the oldest accounts of legal medicine still surviving is a handbook that was written in China in 1250 A.D. It contains information on how to examine bodies, along with descriptions of wounds and directions on how to tell if the wounds were inflicted by sharp or blunt instruments. There is also instruction of determining if victims found in water were drowned or were dead beforehand. Similar information is presented for dealing with victims of fire.

Early immigrants from England brought to the United States the coroner system that was used in the early 1600s. The first recorded coroner's inquest occurred in 1635 in Plymouth, Massachusetts, where it was determined that John Deacon had died due to starvation and extreme cold. Two years later, the governor of Maryland appointed Thomas Baldridge to serve as sheriff and coroner. Soon Baldridge held an inquest concerning the body of John Bryant. The verdict rendered was: ". . . John Bryant by the fall of a tree had his blood bulke broken; and hath two scratches under his chinne on the left side; and so that by means of the fall of the said tree upon him the said John Bryant came to his death."

As early as 1647, autopsy reports of bodies were recorded in Massachusetts. But the earliest formal system requiring American doctors to work with the law was established in 1860 in Maryland, where the Code of Public General Law stated that a physician was required to be present during examination in all cases of violent death.

By 1890, the science of pathology was an important part of forensic medicine in America. The city of Baltimore, Maryland, authorized the Board of Health to appoint two doctors as medical examiners. They were to perform autopsies requested by the coroner. In 1915, New York City created the medical examiner system, which was set up to examine all sudden deaths. Dr. Charles Norris was given authorization to order autopsies when he deemed it necessary. Thus a scientific medical examiner system came into being.

The first state medical examiner system was estabished in Maryland in 1939. Prior to this, the Harvard Medical School in Cambridge, Massachusetts, started teaching legal medicine. Other schools followed suit in later years, and the training program for young pathologists was created and developed.

State police and criminal investigators attend

various schools for short-term courses that teach them how to apply pathology and medical science when investigating violent crimes. Today there are state police laboratories throughout the United States, as well as laboratories in counties and large cities. The Federal Bureau of Investigation and other branches of the federal and state governments use medicine and other sciences to learn the truth about criminal cases.

FBI LABORATORY

The first FBI scientific crime laboratory was set up in the early 1930s. It was founded to fill the special needs of the FBI agents in the field. One unique feature of the FBI system was that each lab examiner received the same training that the field agents got, whether the examiner was an electronics engineer, a physicist, or chemist.

This was important and paid off in ideas that improved performance. For example, it was common knowledge that if a cornered criminal knew he was surrounded, with no possibility of escape, then he might be inclined to give up without bloodshed. But the field agents often had no way of communicating with the criminal without getting too close and thus endangering themselves. The FBI Laboratory was given the problem. The lab scientists solved it by developing a battery-powered, portable amplifier that is capable of sending an agent's voice hundreds of yards. These portable amplifiers are now commonly used not only by FBI agents but by a variety of people, including boat owners and officials supervising track meets.

As important as the FBI Laboratory is today, it is a facility that was slow in coming. Even in the 1920s there was little use of scientific techniques to aid law enforcement in the United States. Concentration at that time was in handwriting analysis or identification; but even so, there were few experts around in the early 1920s. When J. Edgar Hoover, who was then the assistant director of the FBI, called for a list of handwriting experts to be compiled, the resulting list was quite short.

A MEMBER OF THE
FBI LABORATORY.

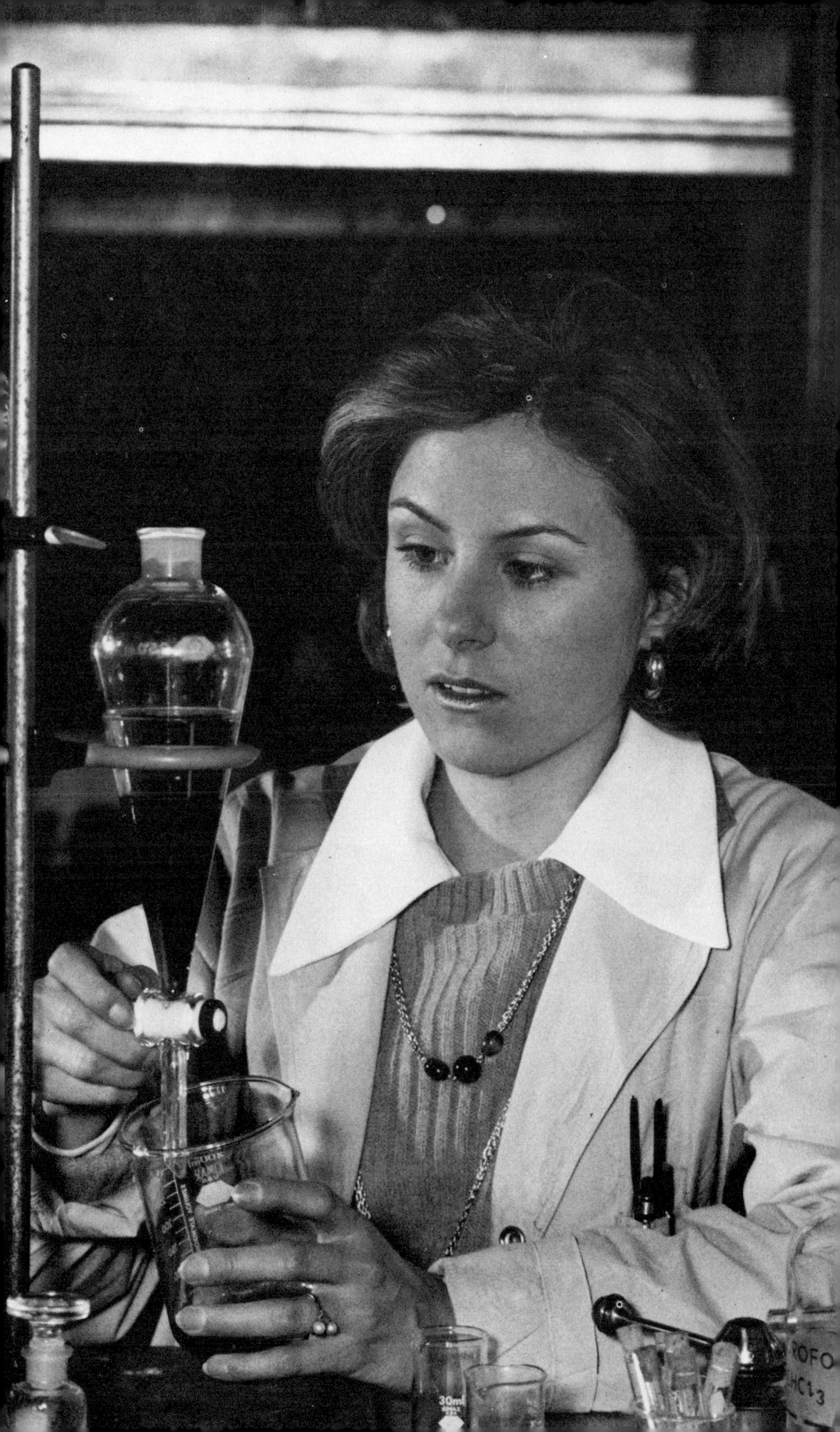
30ml

By 1929, the FBI began assembling a library of books dealing with scientific subjects that related to crime, such as the testing of hair, blood, and various drugs. A strange criminal act played a major part in starting the whole move toward scientific investigation in Chicago—a gangland shooting commonly called the St. Valentine's Day Massacre.

On February 14, 1929, several members of a gang ruled by Al Capone disguised themselves as police and shot and killed seven persons in a garage. The Chicago police kept the bullets they found in the garage after the slayings, and during the trial the police told how they felt they could identify the gun the bullets had been fired from, except that they had no crime laboratory in which to do the work. This bit of information was of great interest to two of the jurors on the coroner's jury. Later, the two jurors helped finance a laboratory in Chicago that became known as the Northwestern University Crime Laboratory.

Hoover heard of the Northwestern University laboratory and other private crime labs as well, and he sent FBI agents to Chicago to study them. As a result the FBI Laboratory was officially opened in November of 1932. Today the multimillion-dollar laboratory is the world's finest-equipped scientific facility for criminal investigation. It is actually an institution for all law enforcement agencies, as it services police laboratories and offices throughout the United States with no charge by examining physical evidence and making identifications of people, chemicals, paint specimens, firearms, and so on.

The fact that the FBI does not charge a fee for its services originally caused complaints from private crime laboratories, which were losing business from the police departments. But Hoover responded to the complaints by claiming that the free laboratory work was payment in kind for help the local police gave the FBI.

FBI scientists have worked at simplifying scientific language so that it can be clearly understood in the courtroom. And the lab has grown so large that the one-room affair of 1932 is now divided into a number of sections. The electronics section develops radio communications. The scientific analysis section deals with the testing of fibers, hairs, blood, poisons, metals, firearms, and more. The documents section is concerned with analyzing forgeries, inks, papers, all kinds of documents, and all kinds of writing, whether by hand, typewriter, printing, or otherwise. The special projects section provides graphic presentations and photographic processing.

The FBI Laboratory also contains huge reference files. Among the items on file are 50,000 different watermarks of paper and thousands of samples of paint, especially from automobiles, to aid identification in hit-and-run cases. Animal hairs, type specimens from the typewriters sold in the United States, and sample tire prints are other items logged in great detail and kept on file.

The laboratory also has a soft X-ray diffractometer that can bombard a substance with X-rays. By studying the angle of the rays, lab scientists can identify any substance without damaging or destroying the substance.

Human hair is one of the most important substances used in investigation. The FBI Laboratory has studied human hair to a great extent and has developed tests that make it possible to tell where the hair may have come from. It is possible to tell from what part of the body a single hair has come, and a single hair can also reveal a person's race and give a hint to the person's age and sex. The lab can also tell if the hair is real or artificial, if it

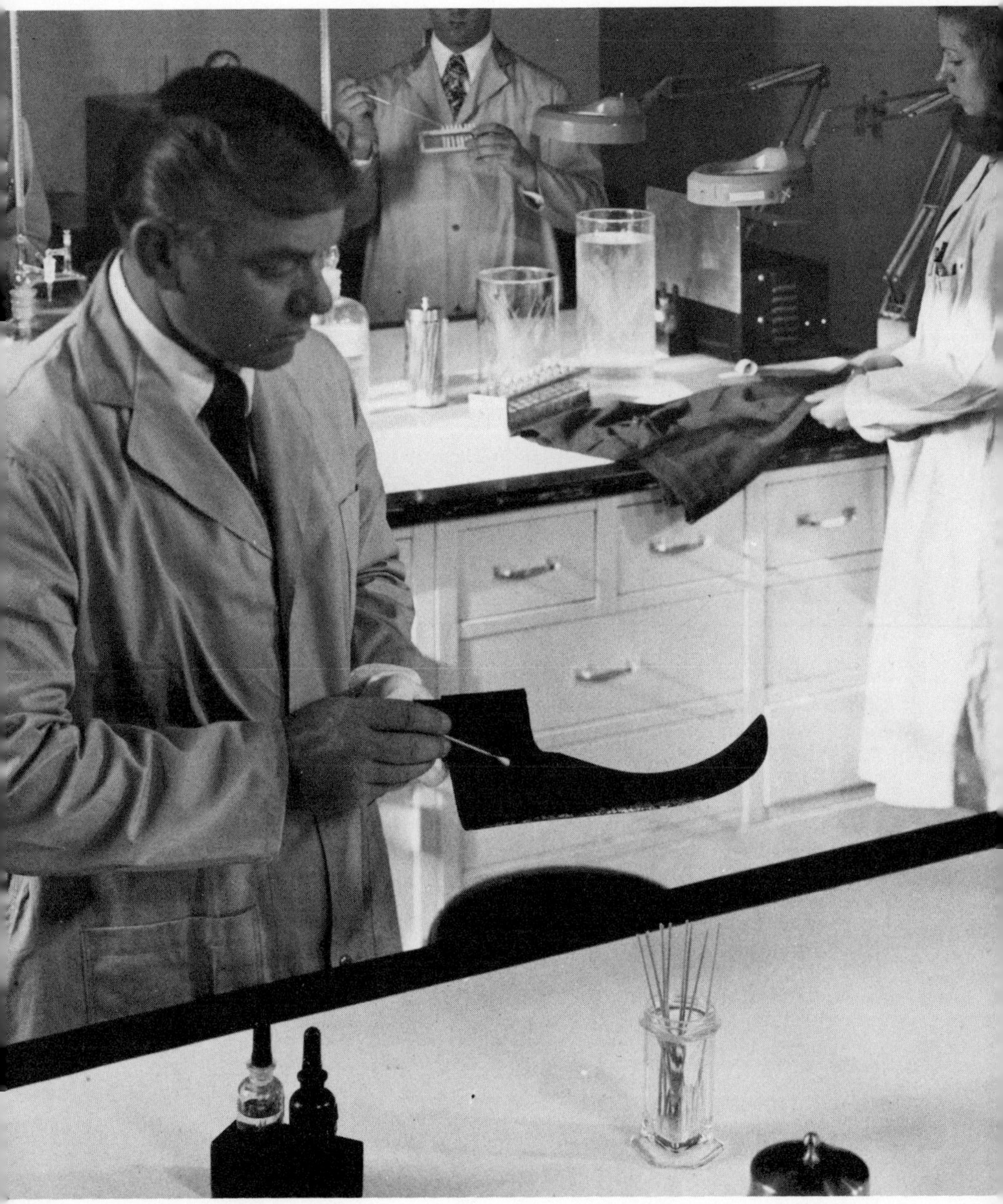

is natural or bleached or dyed, and how the hair was cut or if it was pulled out.

Not only is the lab important in identifying the guilty, but it is equally important in protecting the innocent. Oftentimes in a case the evidence points strongly to one person. This person may claim to be innocent, but the police are forced to go on what they find. The lab can, and often does, show that the person claiming innocence is indeed telling the truth. For example, a hunter in Alaska was found near a dead man. The hunter's socks were covered with blood and he was carrying a recently fired rifle. The dead man had been shot with a rifle. The hunter claimed innocence, but he appeared very guilty. He was cleared, however, when a ballistics test proved that his rifle was not the murder weapon and a chemical test showed that the blood on his socks was from a chicken.

THE SEROLOGY UNIT OF THE FBI LABORATORY SEARCHES FOR BLOOD IN VARIOUS PIECES OF EVIDENCE.

THE CRIME LAB

When a crime is suspected, the police bring in the medical examiner. Once his or her report is in, the police will begin to move if there is evidence suggesting foul play. In the case of any death, of course, there must be an identification of the body. This is usually a simple matter of checking papers found on the body, or comparing photographs, or personal identification by a relative, friend, or coworker. In the case of Dr. Morgan and his wife, identification was made by Amanda Hale, the maid.

As mentioned, lab scientists removed all kinds of physical evidence from the Morgan's bedroom and took the evidence to the DePault crime laboratory. At the laboratory, work was begun to try and learn who shot Dr. Morgan and his wife. This was only after the medical examiner had determined that the case was a double murder and not a murder-suicide.

One of the first items thoroughly examined was the gun. In various tests, such as firing the weapon, the crime lab wanted to make sure it was the gun responsible for the murders. Also, the lab wanted to determine the condition of the gun, if it was fired recently, and from what direction. Also, they wanted to find out whether by some chance the gun could have been fired accidentally. All bullets found at the scene and taken from the bodies were examined, as well as the bullet cartridges.

The murder gun was identified as a .38 caliber snub-nosed revolver. The gun identification number was recorded, and a tracing was begun. All guns sold in the

PHOTOGRAPHS TAKEN AT
THE SCENE ARE LATER
TURNED OVER TO THE LAB.

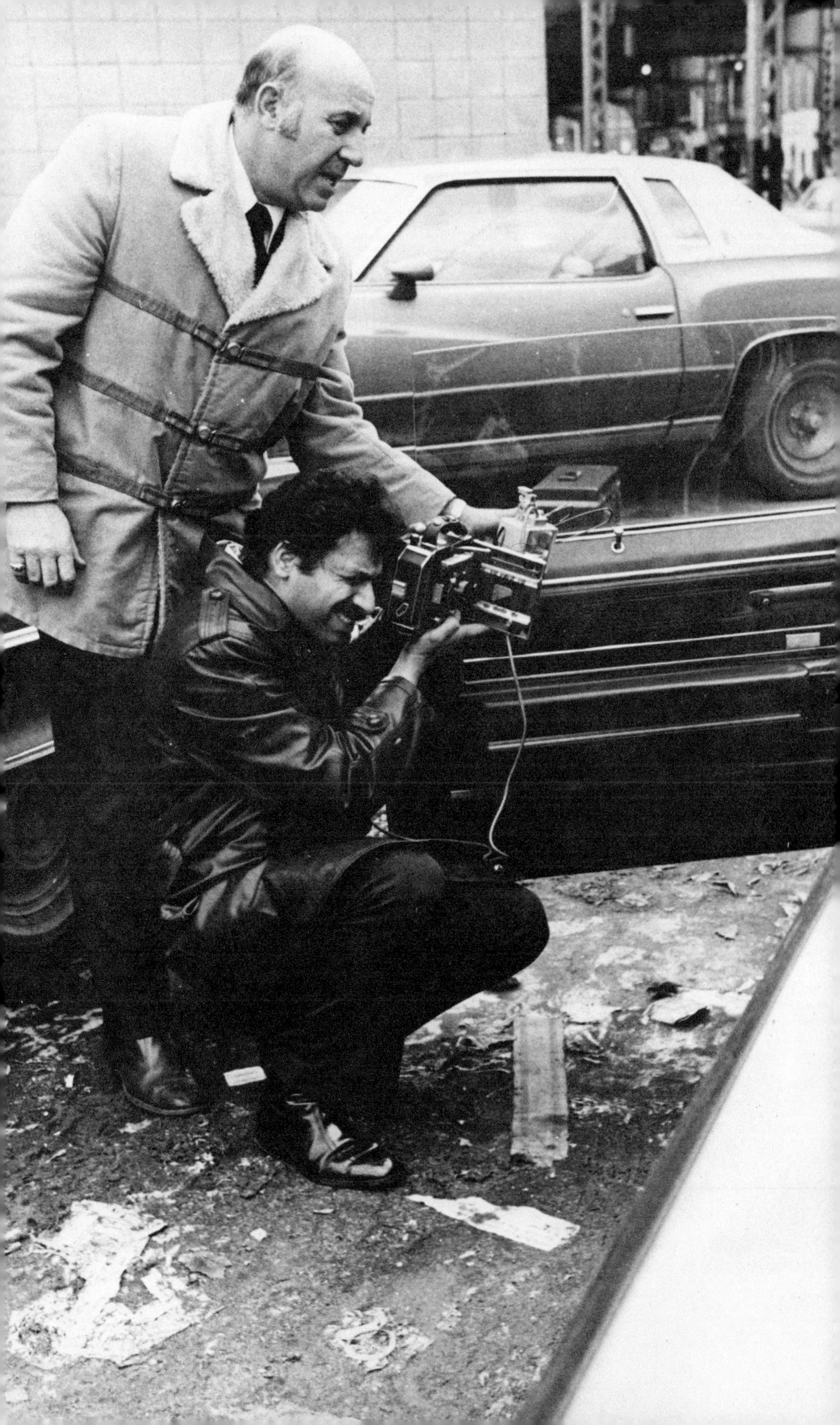

United States have identification numbers recorded by the sellers, and this information is kept on file at police stations. This allows the gun to be traced. When the police found the owner of the .38, he said he had sold the gun several months earlier to a man called Ken. Since there was no further registration, the man was in trouble, but the police wanted to know who the man Ken was. Did he know where Ken lived? The man said he thought Ken was a bartender in the lounge of the Hamilton Hotel. They found Ken at the bar. At first Ken denied ever owning the gun, but when the police told Ken that there was a double murder involved, he admitted he once had owned the gun, but had recently sold it to a customer in the bar. Ken didn't know the man's name. He said the man had offered him a hundred dollars cash for the gun, so he took it . . . no questions asked.

During testing at the lab, the gun was fired into a water-filled tank, from which the bullets were then extracted and examined. During firing, bullets spin rapidly because of grooves in the barrel of the gun. This spinning helps the bullet take a true track as a projectile. However, this grooving leaves marks on the bullet. Because each gun is different, the marks left on each bullet are different. No two guns produce the same marks, so the police can make positive identification of a gun by studying bullets fired from it. They can say for sure that the bullets found in the Morgan's bedroom were from the gun found on the floor. This test is called a ballistics test or firearms examination. It is one of the most common tests performed in a crime lab.

The hairs found in the Morgan bedroom were also examined. There are approximately 120,000 hairs on the average human head. It was reasonable to expect that the hairs found in the bedroom could be from the victims.

But all hairs had to be checked. The color of the hair is noted, as is the makeup, such as the external sheath (or cuticle), the medulla (the central core), and the cortex (the layer that surrounds the medulla). The diameter of human hair varies, as does the shape of the cross-section. The cross-section may be kidney-shaped, triangular, oval, or circular. These shapes and other peculiarities allow the crime scientists, or criminologists, to tell if the hair is from an Indian, Black, Oriental, or Caucasian. The sex and approximate age of the person from which the hair came can also be determined in certain cases.

Lab men and women also found several fingerprints in the Morgan bedroom. Some were easily seen, such as those on the dressing-room table. For others they dusted, using a fingerprint brush and some fine powder of various tones. By dusting with powder, fingerprints can be made to show up on smooth surfaces. The criminologists found some prints on the bureau drawers, on the bedposts, on door handles, and one set on the painted casing near the door. They also took the Morgan's hairbrushes to the lab because they knew they would have fingerprints on the handles. Although the criminologists were certain they wouldn't find any foreign prints on the hairbrushes, they didn't want to overlook anything, or be accused later of not being thorough. The prints were actually lifted off the surfaces by using a sticky tape that is carefully placed over the dusted print. The powdered print is then lifted off the surface and attached to a file card for permanent keeping.

Back at the lab, the scientists would attempt to check the prints with those of Dr. Morgan and his wife. Their fingerprints were taken, as well as those of the maid. If the scientists could not immediately identify

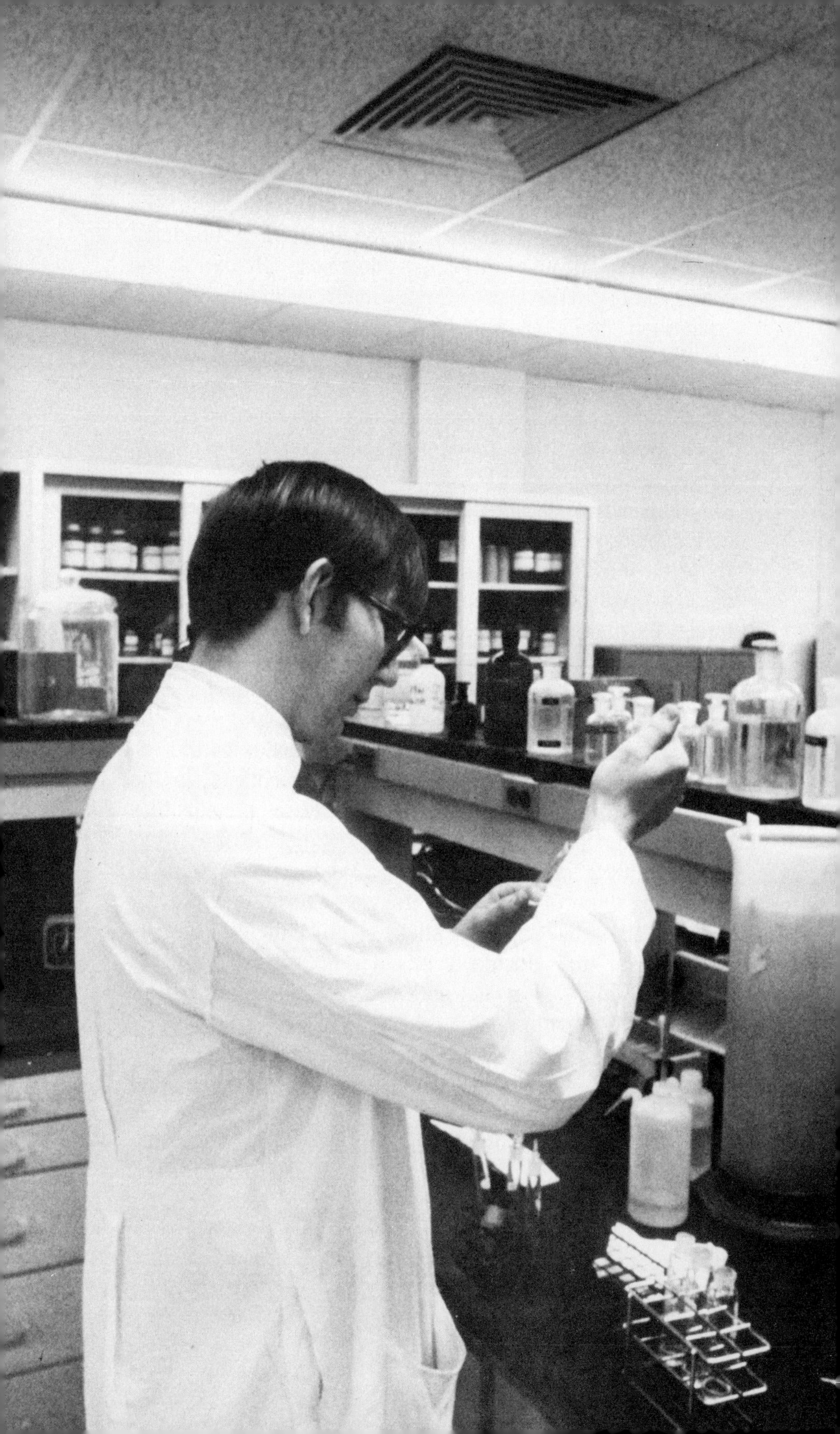

any prints found in the bedroom, they would look into their own police files to attempt to make identification. If they had no luck there, then a copy of the fingerprints and a list of suspects would be sent to the FBI identification division. The FBI Laboratory has more than 170 million prints on file and identifies nearly 2 million sets of prints each year.

Fingerprints have three basic patterns. There are whorl patterns, loops, and arches. The prints are kept on file according to certain classifications. The patterns may be further divided into subgroups. For example, there are plain arches and tented arches; radial loops and ulnar loops; and more. The sets of fingerprints in the FBI files are those of criminals as well as military personnel, applicants for various licenses, aliens, government personnel, and others.

The DePault lab was able to match up fingerprints found at the scene with those of Dr. Morgan and his wife, and with those of Amanda Hale. But they also found a good set of prints from two fingers and a thumb of the left hand on the door casing by the bedroom door. They were fresh prints and they were not on file in the DePault lab, so a copy of the set was sent to the FBI identification division.

The dust taken from the carpet of the bedroom was examined by X-ray to determine what it was and from where it had come. The dust was found to be tiny bits of metal and paint. The paint was automobile paint, so lab personnel said it could be dust from an automobile repair

LAB TECHNICIANS DO
MUCH OF THE ANALYSES.

garage. Other smudges substantiated that theory when they proved to be oil and grease.

The lab investigators returned to the house that had been sealed shut and searched for more dust tracings near the front and back doors and on the stairs leading up to the bedroom. They found what they were looking for. And when more tests were completed, they too indicated that the dust was from paint and metal and that the smudge marks were oil and grease.

After tests on the hair were completed, it was learned there were several hairs from the victims. Other hairs found at the scene belonged to a middle-aged blond woman, later identified as Amanda Hale. Some were dog hairs; the Morgans had owned a dog. And one single, unidentified hair was from some other white person.

The gun was reexamined. The first examination revealed the doctor's fingerprints on the weapon. But now the crime lab people discovered there were minute traces of oil and grease all over the gun. Further tests showed that the grease and oil could be from an oily rag—the kind used by automobile mechanics—although this was not definitely proved.

Police Detective Frank Rogers was given all the new information. Immediately, he began to inquire as to the connection an automobile mechanic might have with the murdered doctor. The maid was able to tell Detective Rogers that one of the doctor's automobiles was to have

THE ATOMIC ABSORPTION SPECTROPHOTOMETER HAS THE ABILITY TO ANALYZE AND IDENTIFY TINY AMOUNTS OF EVIDENCE.

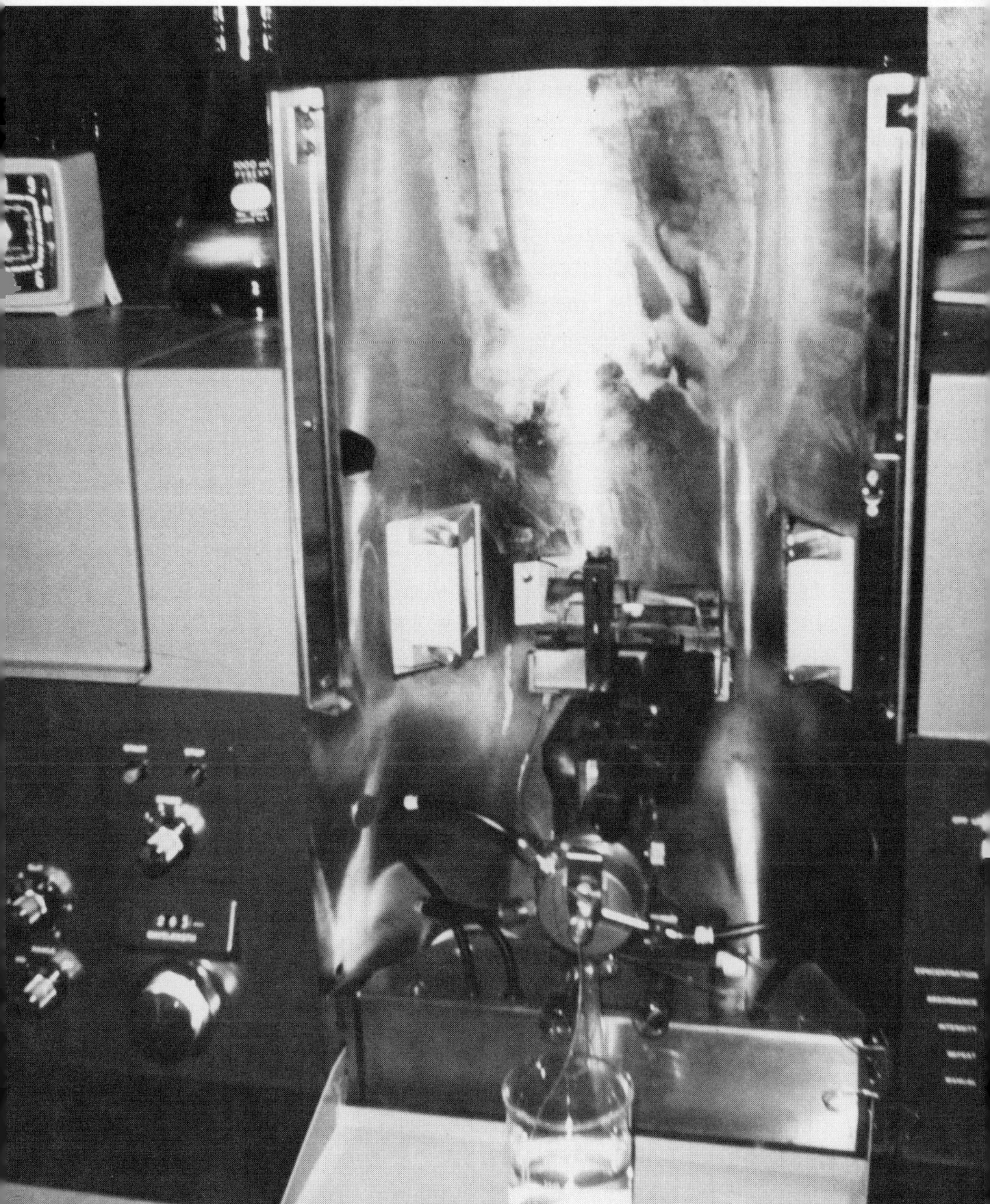

been delivered to the home early in the morning on the day of the murder. The auto had been in a garage for repairs. A visit to the garage where the automobile had been repaired led to the discovery of the identity of the man who delivered the automobile. He was black-haired, Caucasian, and thirty-three years old.

Despite their suspicions, the police still had no case. The crime lab had more work to do. The name of the man who delivered the automobile was sent to the FBI to determine if his fingerprints were in the FBI files, and if so, whether the prints matched any that were found in the bedroom.

Further tests were also made. Bloodstains and other stains found on the carpet and bedding were examined. The blood was found to belong to the victims. There was no blood from anyone else. The stains were from coffee that could have been spilled by anyone. It must be pointed out that the duties of the crime lab are to learn exactly what happened in the bedroom, who was there, and who fired the weapon. It is not the duty of the crime lab to try and find evidence that the auto mechanic was the murderer. He may have been. Or he may have gone to the room, seen the bodies, become frightened, and run away. The crime lab personnel or detectives must examine all evidence. By trying to concentrate on one party or suspect, they may overlook additional clues or evidence that could lead to someone else, perhaps even the actual murderer.

One of the particles found in the bedroom was what is commonly called lint. The crime lab scientists believed it came from a pocket. They examined tiny threads and identified the color, length, and twist of the thread. They were able to tell the type of material the thread had come from. In time, they found extremely tiny bits of the same material on the murder gun.

Upon questioning the garage mechanic, the police also took his fatigue jacket so that it could be examined by the crime lab. After examination of the material in the pocket, the scientists determined that the gun had been in the pocket of the jacket. They were able to compare the threads and could state that the jacket had definitely been in the bedroom. Now the case was firming up.

Later, the FBI report on the fingerprints came in. The FBI was able to provide identification because the man from the auto repair shop had served in the Army. When Detective Rogers learned of the latest developments, he obtained an arrest order and the garage mechanic was brought into custody. The mechanic admitted he delivered the automobile, but he claimed he had walked right back to the garage and returned to work. However, Frank Rogers began offering the proof obtained by the crime lab. The suspect's fingerprints were found in the room. Threads from his fatigue jacket were found on the floor of the bedroom and on the murder weapon. And the police would be able to offer the testimony of the man named Ken who had sold the gun to the suspect.

Faced with all this crime lab evidence and the testimony of Ken the bartender, the mechanic confessed to the double murder of the doctor and his wife. After delivering the automobile, the mechanic had entered the back door with robbery in mind. He had heard that the doctor's wife had an expensive collection of jewelry. Upstairs, the mechanic discovered the doctor and his wife asleep. He searched the bureau drawers for the jewel case, but suddenly the doctor awoke and challenged him. He knew both could identify him, so the mechanic first shot the doctor and then killed the wife while she was in bed. He tried to make the killings look like suicide and murder, and he almost succeeded.

Later, the jewel box was discovered in the mechanic's locker at the repair garage. And as far as Detective Rogers was concerned, the crime was solved.

ARSON

There are other crimes not as easily solved. One such crime is arson. Arson—the deliberate, malicious setting of a destructive fire—is not an uncommon crime. In fact, it is a crime that is rapidly on the rise. The motive in most cases of arson is money. For example, it is not uncommon for someone to buy a piece of property, such as an apartment building, and put a great deal of insurance on it. The apartment building is rented out, and over the years it deteriorates badly. The cost of fixing the building may be thousands of dollars. And the income from the renting of apartments may be falling off because the building becomes occupied by low-income families who cannot pay much rent. Or local taxes may rise to a point where the apartment owner cannot make any money, and in fact loses money. The apartment owner then sets, or pays someone to set, the building on fire so that the owner can collect full insurance.

For this reason, and many others, all fires are investigated thoroughly to see if the fire was accidental or of suspicious origin. When a fire inspector or fire marshal arrives at the scene of a fire, he or she must ask the following questions. Where and how was the fire started? Was it accidental or on purpose? If suspicious, is there evidence as to how it was started and any clues regarding who was responsible?

A fire marshal realizes that for any fire, regardless if it involves a whole building or just a small fireplace, several things are necessary. There must be something to ignite the fire, such as a candle, match, or something similar. There must be inflammable material, such as papers, gasoline, or cleaning fluid. And there must be a good supply of the inflammable material as well as a free supply of oxygen.

An intentionally set fire quite often is started with

flame, an electrical means, or with chemicals or acid. Accidental fires are the result of an almost endless variety of causes—a cigarette, a short circuit in an electrical wire, embers from a fireplace, woodwork near stovepipes, the sun's rays shining through a bottle of liquid, sparks from a controlled fire, an electric torch, and so on.

Unlike the crime lab scientist, who can examine the scene of a crime and then take samples back to the laboratory for more analysis, the fire marshal must spend most of his or her time at the fire scene. The fire expert will first take statements from witnesses in an attempt to discover when and where the fire started. Usually, the spot where the fire originated shows signs of the most intense heat and for the longest time. It also has the most charring of wood or melting of glass and metal. But this is not always the case. Sometimes there may be some highly combustible material elsewhere that ignited, causing a hotter fire someplace away from where the fire originated.

Fire marshals try to learn from witnesses when smoke first came from a building. If the building is empty then they want to know the time the last person left. They want to know where it starts, why, and if it was accidental. They want to know how much of the woodwork is burned and how deep. Common woodwork burns at the rate of an inch and a half per hour. Was the fire smoldering? Are there smoke stains on windows or walls? These are all things taken into consideration by the fire inspector to determine if there is arson involved.

If a burning cigarette or carelessly tossed lit match caused a fire, there will be no evidence of that fact at the scene. If the fire was caused by a faulty heater or some other means such as an electrical appliance, then the fire inspector can get a pretty good idea of how the fire started, because when the fire is localized so is the damage.

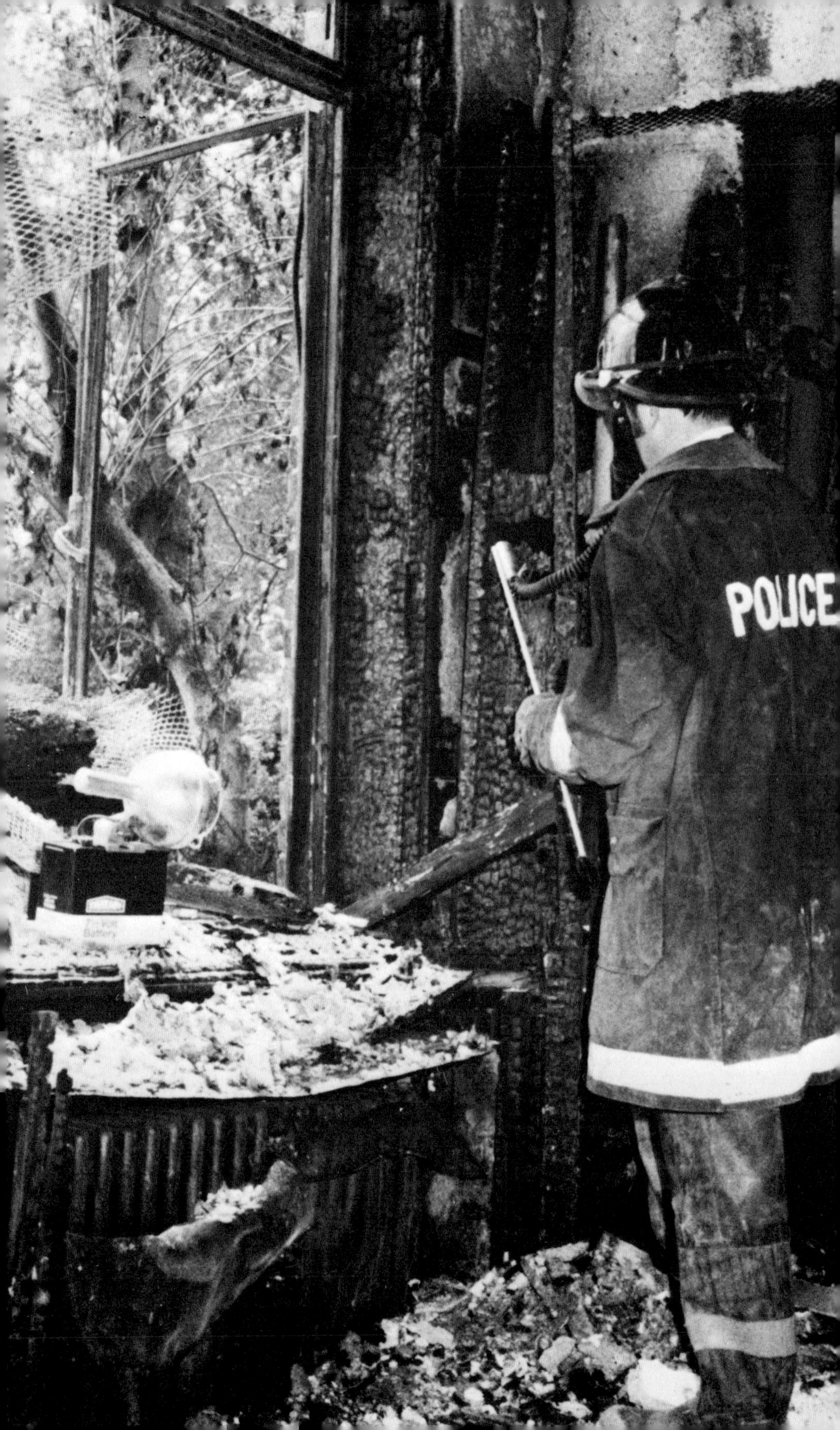
POLICE

In one particular case involving a fire of suspicious origin, the fire inspector found a small electric heater in a country inn that had just burned to the ground. Close examination revealed that the heater had been just as hot inside as it was on the outside. This made the fire inspector curious. If the heater had just been subjected to an ordinary fire, it would only be damaged on the outside, and not on the inside as well. This led the investigator to ask the inn's guests certain questions. After much examination and questioning, it was learned that the heater had been packed with highly inflammable material and that it had been left turned on. However, the fuses in the fuse box had been removed. The fire inspector learned that when the inn guests found no lights, they did the natural thing and went to the fuse box. By replacing the fuses, the guests turned on the heater, which ignited the materials packed inside of it, and started a fire. The inn owner was confronted with the evidence and soon confessed to what he thought was a foolproof crime of arson.

When inspecting a fire, the fire marshal must always be aware that the fire could have been started not only by an arsonist, but by a pyromaniac, someone who sets fires because he or she enjoys it. In cases suspected of involving a pyromaniac, the fire marshal asks if there have been other fires in the building or area. Does the same person turn in the alarm? If simple arson is suspected, he or she may ask if the building has high insurance?

ARSON INVESTIGATION
BEGINS AS SOON AS THE
AREA IS SAFE TO ENTER.

Is the owner in financial straits? Have small, suspicious fires destroyed records only, or large sums of money? Have two of more fires broken out at the same time? And have inflammable materials been found at the scene that really shouldn't be there?

These questions were applied to a book barn fire that seemed suspicious. The owner, in need of money, was out of town at the time of the fire. The fire destroyed the building and all of the books. And the fire inspector found that the building was covered by a great deal of insurance. So the fire inspector looked for anything unusual—something that ordinarily wouldn't be found along with thousands of books. He found the remains of a plastic wading pool—the kind used by small children in the summer. A plastic wading pool isn't an item likely to be found in a book barn. There was also a glass candle holder, cracked and broken, probably from extreme heat. Further investigation and questioning of the book barn owner revealed that the fire had been set. The wading pool had been filled with an inflammable liquid, enough to submerge the candle holder. Then the candle was placed into the holder and carefully lit. The book barn owner then left town. Slowly the candle burned down, until it reached the liquid. The result was an instant fire and a solid excuse for the owner of the book barn. But hard work by the fire inspector didn't allow the owner to get away with the crime.

If the book barn owner hadn't finally admitted what he had done, there were other methods the fire marshal could have used to try and build a case establishing that the fire was arson. Samples of the debris of the fire can be taken to a laboratory. In the case of the book barn, burned books could be examined. Using steam distillation techniques, scientists can find residues of paint thinners, kerosene, gasoline, or alcohol. This method is not foolproof, but if traces of kerosene are found on the burned books, then the fire marshal can search the premises for containers of kerosene or check on sales of kerosene to the suspect. With hard work, cases against arsonists can be made.

THE FORENSIC DENTIST

Dr. Morgan and his wife were easy to identify. Their maid, Amanda Hale, just had to view the faces of the bodies to make it certain. But in cases of major accidents, such as a fire or an airplane crash, the forensic dentist is called upon to identify victims so badly burned or mutilated that they cannot otherwise be recognized.

For centuries dentistry was used in identification. One well-known practitioner of dentistry was Paul Revere, who, during the American Revolution, identified the bodies of British and Colonial officers by the very teeth he had worked on when they were alive.

In identification the dentist may use either the jaw of the deceased or complete dental charts. Then the dental chart from the victim's dentist is examined. When the charts compare or are similar, then a very complete study is made. Eventually, identification is almost certain.

Identification can be positive because there are enough distinctive characteristics of teeth to make identification almost a sure thing. Each person has five dental surfaces on as many as 32 teeth, which leaves a total of 160 surfaces. Then there are missing teeth, decayed surfaces, fillings, rotated teeth, teeth out of line, false teeth, variations of arch, and other visible features to give an almost indefinite number of characteristics. It is safe to say that, with enough information about a person's teeth, those teeth will prove to be unlike any other persons.

Only recently has it been realized that dental information distinguishes a person's teeth and makes them equally as unique as fingerprints. Just since 1967 have

FORENSIC DENTISTRY HAS BECOME AN IMPORTANT AID TO IDENTIFICATION.

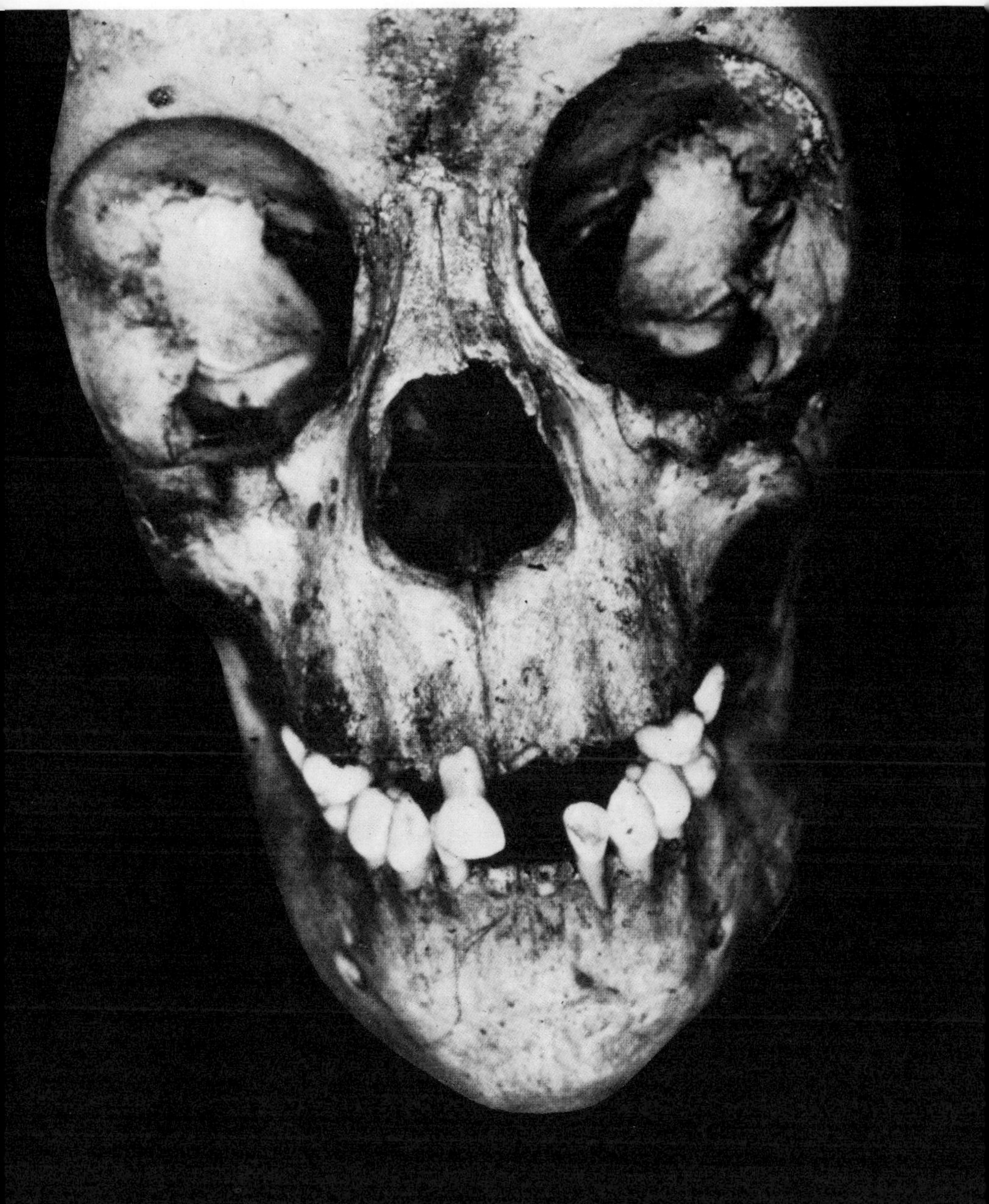

the courts in a few states allowed the admission of bite marks as evidence in criminal cases. Such states as Maryland, Illinois, Texas, California, Florida, New York, and Connecticut have already allowed forensic dentists to testify.

For example, in a recent murder case in Maryland a suspect pleaded innocent. He was examined by a well-known forensic dentist. An impression was taken of the defendant's teeth and was compared to photographs of teeth marks found on the body of the murder victim. Identification was positive and the man was convicted.

Because it has already proved valuable in solving a number of crimes, forensic dentistry is likely to be used more and more. In the beginning, there were few people trained to even see bite marks on victims. It is often difficult for the untrained eye to recognize bite marks because they can be easily confused with other bruises.

Bite marks are not as reliable as fingerprints but they do give a good idea of who did the biting—or, at the very least, who did *not* do the biting. Trained forensic dentists can see bite marks on the skin and, after examination, tell if they were made by an attacker, by a victim of an attack, or during close encounters such as love-making. Also, it can be generally determined when the bite mark was made and the position of the bodies during the attack. This kind of information is essential when police are trying to corroborate the testimony of a defendant or a witness. Through the testimony of a forensic dentist, defendants can be convicted or acquitted.

In one case in New York, the defendant stated that he was bitten by an attacker, so he killed the attacker as an act of self-defense. However, a forensic dentist who studied the bite marks testified that the bite marks were made at an earlier date and could not have been made by the dead man. The defendant was forced to change his story and was later convicted of murder.

It is believed that the first *major* case in which a court allowed evidence centered on bite marks occurred in 1973 in Illinois. A forensic dentist testified that bite marks found on a dead woman could not have been made by the man who was the defendant in the case. The dentist stated that the defendant's teeth were not the same size as the bite marks and that the arch of the man's mouth did not match the arch that would be necessary to produce the marks. At first, the man was convicted anyway, because this was the first time for bite-mark testimony. However, new evidence was uncovered later to prove that the forensic dentist was absolutely correct. A new trial ensued, and the man was found not guilty.

In one of the strangest of bite-mark cases, bite marks on the victim were not discovered at the time of the postmortem examination by the pathologist. The bite marks were not found until two years later, when a forensic dentist was studying photographs of the victim.

The body was exhumed (brought up) from the grave to be reexamined. Because of a good embalming, the body was in top condition. The dentist was able to determine that the bite marks had been cut with a knife at the time of the murder in order to disguise them. And the cover-up had almost worked.

A further complication in this bizarre case arose when it was discovered that the teeth of the prime suspect, who had been let go, had been removed since the murder. The dentist got around this obstacle by using a special computer microscope to compare the bite marks to old X-rays of the man's teeth. The bite marks matched up with the suspect's teeth, and the result was a belated conviction.

NAPOLEON TEST

The marvelous scientific instruments found in modern crime laboratories have other uses. They are not just used to solve crimes.

One interesting example of the use of crime instruments in a historical case involves thin strands of hair with tiny, invisible protons to try and answer a question that is often asked: What or who killed the French emperor Napoleon?

A team of scientists from the Massachusetts Institute of Technology has been working with nine hairs belonging to Napoleon. The goal is to learn if the famous French emperor was, as is suggested in some historical accounts, poisoned with arsenic. To date, the answer is not clear. After all, Napoleon died more than 150 years ago. But it is interesting to know that this type of investigation can be done and that it can be done with a degree of success, even if the answer cannot be stated with 100 percent accuracy.

A scientist in England supplied the MIT team with the hairs. The English scientist had read that the hairs could be analyzed by means of new techniques involving bombardment with protons. He wrote a letter to the MIT team and asked if they would do the study. The thinking was that if the MIT scientists could rule out arsenic as the cause of death, then the other possibility was that Napoleon died of stomach cancer.

The MIT team was interested in the matter because in history there have been countless papers written and published stating that Napoleon died of arsenic poisoning and nothing else. But some historians are not so sure that this is positively accurate. So the MIT study is underway.

In their study, the MIT scientists have used a powerful instrument known as the proton microprobe which fires protons (elementary atomic particles that are the nuclei of hydrogen atoms) at a sample of the hair. When the protons interact with the atoms in the small section of the hair, electrons from the hair's atoms are knocked out. This produces X-rays that show the same characteristics of arsenic, lead, or mercury. When the scientists read the X-rays, they can actually tell what is in the hair sample. The scientists bombard each individual hair and also look at extremely small sections of each hair to check for the presence of arsenic or, for that matter, anything else.

The scientists have examined all nine hairs and so far they have found arsenic in some of them. But they have also found no traces of arsenic in others. Because of these findings, the scientists cannot say for sure that Napoleon was poisoned and that a crime was committed, or that he wasn't poisoned. One main reason for the uncertain results is that the nine hairs used in the test were not taken from Napoleon's head all at the same time. They were samples gathered at different times of his life. It is thought that the hairs were cut by the emperor and given to his many lady friends as gifts of love or perhaps as a souvenir of some sort. All the hairs were in excellent condition, well dated, and considered to be most precious.

In an earlier study of Napoleon's hair, a process using neutrons was used. These experiments showed that there were arsenic levels in the hair some thirteen times higher than normal. But the scientists who conducted that study stated that even this high amount wasn't enough arsenic to kill the emperor. Besides, it is well known that during Napoleon's period of prominence arsenic was taken internally in small doses by royalty and people of note who considered it a beauty aid. Arsenic, it was believed then, made the skin look pure and translucent and made the hair on the head glossy and sleek.

The very first study on the emperor's hair was done

shortly after his death. The sample used in that study was much larger than the nine hairs examined at MIT. It was done on St. Helena Island in the south Atlantic. But the examiners were unable to learn how much arsenic was in the hair and how the levels differed from one hair to the other. In fact, they couldn't even tell how much arsenic was in one end of the hair compared to the other end.

There was an autopsy made on the body, and its findings are amazing. On the autopsy report, the doctor stated that the emperor died of stomach cancer, not arsenic poisoning. The report also indicated that the emperor had bad teeth, hemorrhoids, constipation, undulant fever, hepatitis, a peptic ulcer, liver inflammations, malaria, dysentery, poor circulation, epilepsy, tuberculosis, pleurisy, hormonal imbalance, syphilis, and gonorrhea. If the report is accurate, Napoleon was a physical wreck and could have died from a number of causes. But perhaps the doctor performing the autopsy, realizing that he was working on a famous man, wanted to show the world he was more than fully qualified.

THE EXPERTS

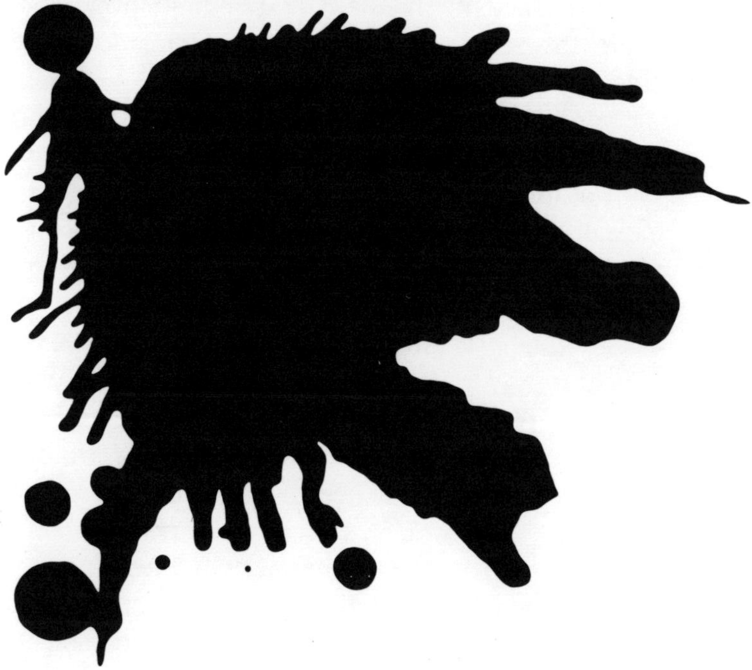

POLYGRAPH EXPERT

Polygraphists are scientists who are coming into more and more prominence in the field of criminal investigation. They are the specialists who give lie detector tests on a machine that is called a polygraph.

The polygraph instrument can tell, to a certain degree of accuracy, whether a person is answering a yes-or-no question with a lie or with the truth. What the instrument does is measure the heartbeat, blood pressure, rate of breathing, and electrical conductivity of the skin (caused by perspiration) during the questioning period.

A person who is willing to take the test (it is not usually mandatory) will be seated in a laboratory. Two rubber tubes are placed around the waist and chest of the subject. The tubes measure the person's rate of breathing. A metal plate is attached to one of the person's hands to measure changes in the rate of perspiration on the skin. A six-inch layer of material with wires inside is wound around and fastened firmly to the arm of the subject. This "cuff," as it is called, measures the person's heartbeat and blood pressure.

Most professional polygraphists are college-educated scientists who have studied courses in psychology. After college, they take a course of several weeks in length to learn how to use the polygraph—not only how to attach the various parts to the subject, but also how to ask questions and then interpret the results.

When the test is begun, the polygraphist starts to ask the questions. The machine traces ink lines on a roll of paper. There are four lines, each representing one of the four measures—heartbeat, blood pressure, breathing rate, and perspiration output on the skin. The paper is constantly moving in the machine as the tracings are made. This allows the polygraphist to easily read the ink tracings.

The polygraphist asks questions that have known true answers, as well as questions pertaining to the particular criminal case. The subject is in a position to prove himself or herself innocent or to reveal that he or she may have some knowledge of the crime. One early question may be, "Is your name John Roberts?" If the man is John Roberts and he answers in the affirmative, then the lines are noted as the condition of the suspect when speaking a true answer. Later, a question about the crime may be asked. "Did you own a .38 caliber revolver?" If there are differences in the ink lines on the paper, then there may be reason to suspect that John Roberts is not telling the truth. Dozens of questions can be asked. The result is a pattern that the polygraphist will be able to decipher. This will tell the lie detector expert if the person being tested is answering truthfully or falsely.

The results of the polygraph test cannot be used in most courtrooms. But the police can use the polygraph to more quickly release innocent people and concentrate their investigations on those who may actually have been involved.

FIREARMS EXPERT

Large crime laboratories usually have a firearms expert. He or she has knowledge of most, if not all, of the firearms that have been manufactured. This expert's specialty is most important because a great many of the violent crimes committed in the United States involve the use of a firearm.

We already know that bullets, through ballistics tests, can be matched, allowing exact identification of a gun used in a crime. But firearms experts can also examine the cartridge shells that held the bullet before firing

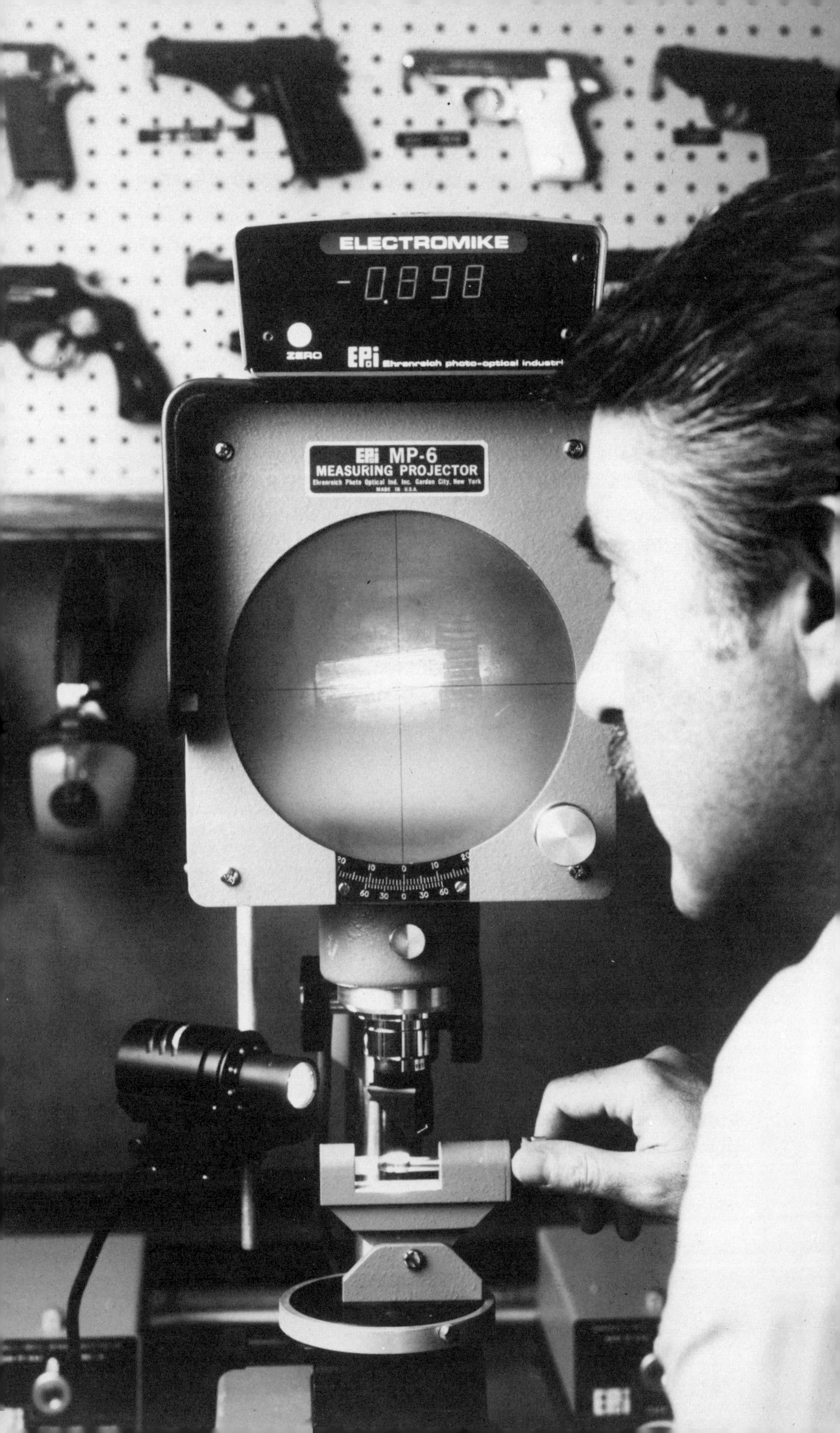
ELECTROMIKE
-0.898
ZERO
EPi Ehrenreich photo-optical industri
EPi MP-6
MEASURING PROJECTOR
Ehrenreich Photo Optical Ind. Inc. Garden City, New York
MADE IN U.S.A.

and make a match. A detective may find a cartridge shell at a murder scene, but the bullet itself may be lost. It may have passed right through the victim and become lost in the woods or ended up in the ocean or at the bottom of a lake. It would be impossible to find. In such cases, the firearms expert can still help, and often does.

On the back of a cartridge case is the primer. This is the area that is struck by the gun's firing pin when the trigger is pulled. The firing pin slams into the primer, causing it to explode. This small explosion causes the powder in the cartridge case to explode simultaneously, forcing the bullet out of the case, through the barrel, and into the air with extreme force. The mark left on the cartridge case by the firing pin is as unique as a fingerprint. No two guns produce the same marks. So a match can be made by the firearms expert using an instrument called the comparison microscope, the same instrument used in the ballistics test. The two cartridge cases are placed in the microscope and then they are examined magnified thousands of times. This makes it easy to make a comparison.

Another method that firearms experts use to try and tie a suspect to the scene of a shooting is the wax glove test. When a gun is fired, tiny specks of gunpowder remain on the hand of the person who fires the weapon. To test for traces of this gunpowder, paraffin, a wax, is melted and then brushed onto the hands of a suspect.

THE FIREARMS EXPERT IS EXAMINING THE RIFLING MARKS ON A BULLET FROM A .38 CALIBER REVOLVER.

When the wax hardens, it forms a sort of "wax glove" that can be cut off the hands and examined.

What the expert looks for are two elements in the wax—antimony and barium. By using an instrument that sends out neutrons—invisible particles found in the nucleus of atoms—the expert bombards the wax. This bombardment causes the atoms to become radioactive. When the radioactive material is counted, it can be identified on the basis of the number of rays it emits. If there is antimony or barium in the wax, the pattern of the emitted rays will tell the firearms expert that the elements are there. If a suspect is known to have recently fired a gun, that information will help in the investigation and will certainly keep the suspect on the list of possible criminals.

THE CORONER AND THE AUTOPSY

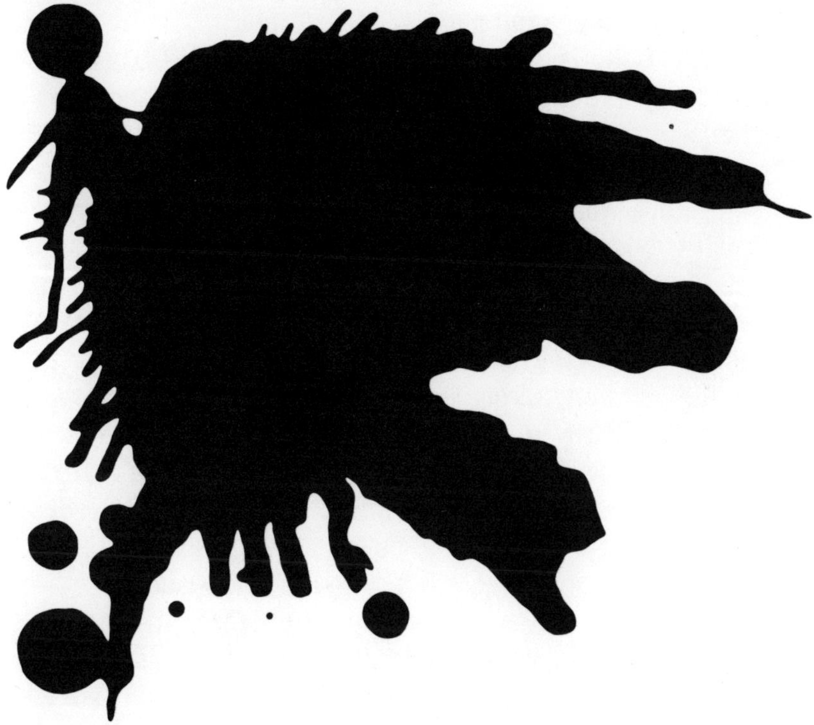

An autopsy is performed to learn how and why a person died, and to determine the time of death. Autopsies may also provide information that allows positive identification of the victim, if the body has not already been identified. In the performance of the autopsy, the coroner is assisted by one or two trained lab technicians. In most cases of suspected crime, a full autopsy is performed.

The body is removed from the rubberized bags and placed on an examination table. All observations are either written down or, as is the case in some laboratories, the findings can be spoken into a microphone and recorded. If there are wounds, photographs are taken, and in most cases the body is X-rayed.

Most bodies are clothed when they are delivered to the coroner. The first thing the coroner does is make a description of the clothing. The clothing is examined carefully, and any foreign matter clinging to it is removed, recorded, and saved. In the case of a gunshot, the coroner would record where the bullet entered. If there was an exit hole from the bullet, that too would be recorded. In order to determine the path of the bullet, any evidence of close-range firing, such as gunpowder, would be measured.

After the clothing has been fully examined, it is carefully removed without cutting or tearing. It is packed in plastic for storage. If it is wet with either water or blood, it will be allowed to dry before storing. All clothes are signed for in the chain of custody.

Once the clothing is taken care of, then the naked body is examined. Physical characteristics, the weight, height, color of hair, scars, and a description of the teeth are recorded. The number and the location of bullet holes are recorded if the victim has been shot. All bruises are noted, as well as wounds of any kind, needle marks, and the like. And a description is made of each wound, noting whether it is round, narrow, or slit-like.

The victim's wounds are examined for fabric fibers and, if it is a gunshot victim, for evidence of gunpowder and bullet fragments. This is important. Later, in test firings, the distance from which the gun was fired can be determined by the residue of soot and gunpowder.

Once all wounds and abrasions are recorded, the body is photographed from all angles. Close-ups are taken of all wounds, cuts, and so on.

If the victim is a gunshot case, then the coroner will trace the path of the bullet. If the bullet or its fragments are still in the body, they will be removed and sent to the crime lab, where a description of the bullet or bullets will be made for the record.

The coroner will open the body by making incisions in the chest. There are usual cuts to be made. The cause of death will then be determined. Was it from severe bleeding? Was it from strangulation? Was it from infection or from pneumonia? Was it from poisoning? Or was it from natural causes?

No matter whether the victim was dead from bleeding or from unknown causes, the coroner will remove the vital organs and liquids from the body. These are removed for further study, especially by the toxicologist.

All urine in the bladder is removed, as well as the contents of the stomach and the bile from the gall bladder. Many drugs concentrate in the gall bladder. One kidney is removed, as is one-half of the liver, one-half of the brain, one lung, a sample of the body fat, heart blood, bone, and hair samples. All are placed in separate containers and labeled. The containers, made of glass or plastic, are sterile. Once the specimens are collected and labeled, they are sealed tight and refrigerated or frozen. Again, each goes through the chain of custody.

When the autopsy is complete, the body is returned to the morgue and is then released to the family of the victim for burial.

THE TOXICOLOGIST

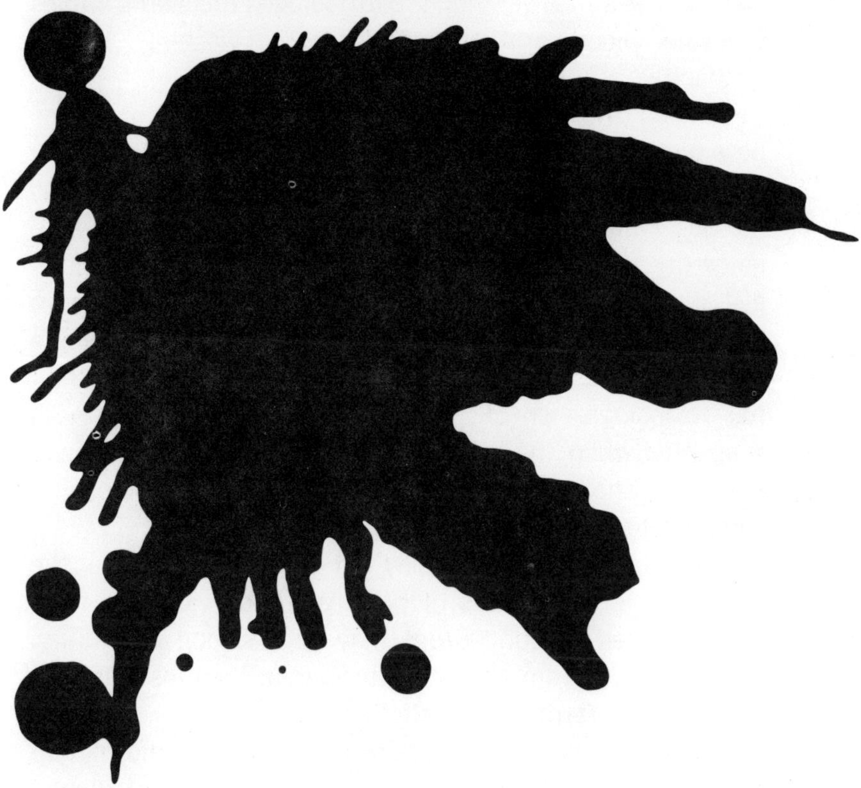

The toxicologist receives and signs for the body organs in the sealed containers. This is for the continuation of the chain of custody. However, if the victim of suspected poisoning is still alive, then the toxicologist receives samples of urine, blood, and any vomit or the washings of the stomach.

Then the toxicologist needs to know as much as possible about the victim, either dead or alive. Information from the investigating police officers is taken, as well as the observations made at the scene by the medical investigator (in the case of a suspected homicide). The toxicologist also wants samples of any household chemicals in the victim's home, such as drugs from the medicine cabinet and pesticides. If sleeping pills are suspected, then the toxicologist checks the victim's liver. If aspirin is suspected, then the victim's urine will be analyzed. Lead poisoning shows up in the bones, and arsenic poisoning can be detected by testing the hair.

Hunches and logic play an important part in the search for certain kinds of poisons. If the victim is from the city, then narcotic drugs may be a strong possibility. If the victim is from an agricultural area, then insecticides, common on a farm, are possibilities.

Also of use to the toxicologist is any information about what the victim ate and drank. And the toxicologist wants to know what symptoms the victim had and when they first occurred. In addition, the toxicologist inquires

THE TOXICOLOGIST EXAMINES
MANY TISSUES TO HELP
DETERMINE CAUSE OF DEATH.

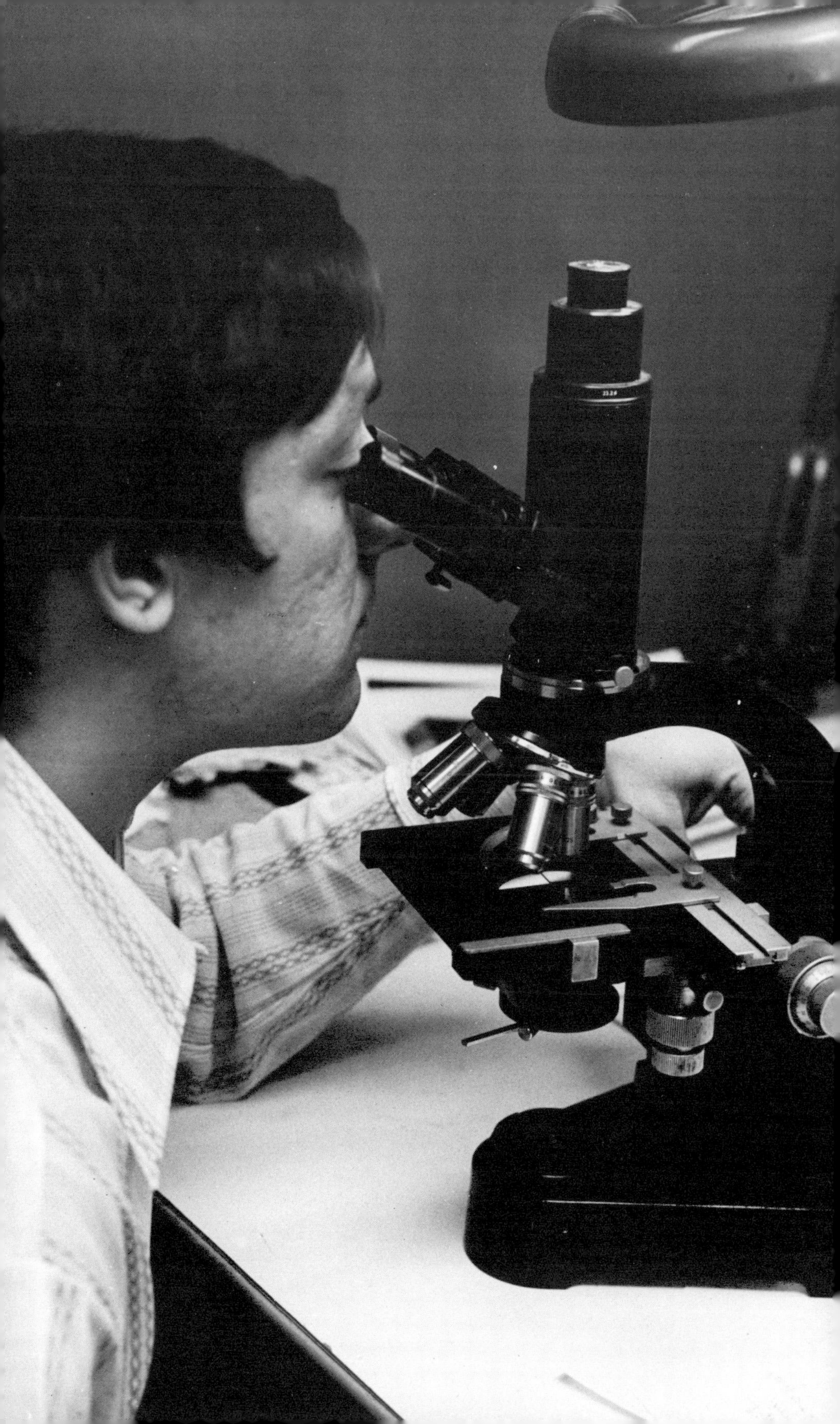

whether the victim received any medical help and whether any antidote was administered.

The spleen, intestines, brain, urine, blood, fat, tissues, and other body elements may be examined to see if there is any trace of a poison strong enough to kill. But in cases where the victim dies several days after taking the poison, the poisonous substance may be out of the body altogether by the time of death. Then the toxicologist must study the organs individually. Often, the organs change because of a poisoning.

During the laboratory examination, the toxicologist makes a chemical analysis of the tissues of the organs and of the liquids, such as blood and urine. There are also tests which evaluate specimens from the body by converting them to gases or steam vapors for analysis. From these tests the toxicologist can determine if any poisons are present in the victim's system.

When the toxicologist engages in his or her laboratory work, portions of the organs and liquids must be saved. Usually, about a third of the available samples are set aside and kept sealed and frozen. This is in case the charge of poisoning ends up in court in which case the defense lawyer may want to have his or her own toxicology expert examine the organs. And the findings may be the same or they may differ.

COMPUTERS IN THE CRIME LAB

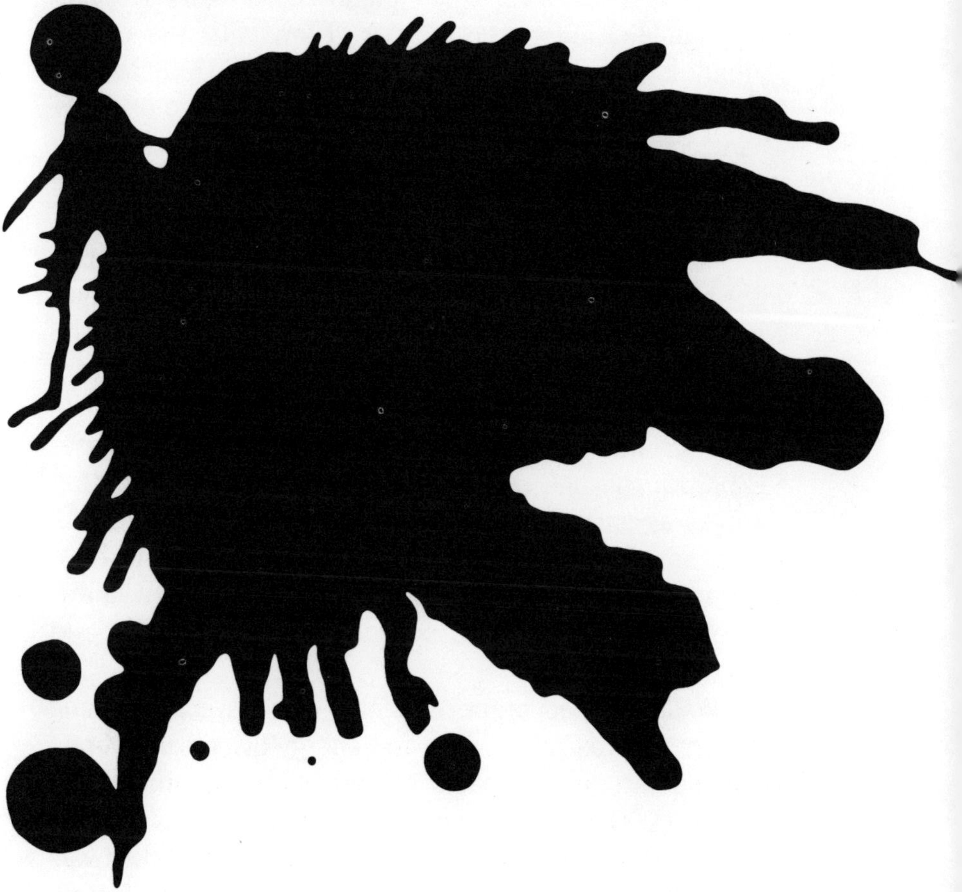

The space age has hit the police laboratories as well as other areas. And it is working in favor of the police and to the disadvantage of the criminal. In New York City, for example, burglary cases involving just a few hundred dollars were often set aside by the police because of the shortage of personnel. The fingerprint department could only handle 1,500 cases a year. Now, with the aid of computers, the fingerprint staff can handle 6,000 cases in a year, and there is promise that the figure will go up. Now when someone reports a burglary of a few hundred dollars the field lab officer can look for fingerprints with the knowledge that there will be a follow-up.

Some of the big-city crime laboratories are equipped with sensitive electronic instruments that can analyze pieces of paint or traces of drugs that are invisible to the naked eye. Some of these devices can find tiny fragments of glass as well. One such instrument is the gas chromatograph-mass spectrometer, a device that costs about $125,000. This unique piece of equipment can analyze drug samples as small as one picogram, or .000,000,000,001 of a gram. Recently, a murder victim was found to have a minute trace of a drug in his body. That trace was evidence enough to link a suspect directly to the crime and get a conviction.

Well-equipped crime labs may also have a scanning electron microscope with an energy-dispersive X-ray. This microscope is capable of very high magnification—up to 40,000 times. In one case a burglar had entered and robbed an apartment, and one of the items taken was the telephone. The phone was yanked from the wall, leaving behind a broken wire. When police found a telephone with broken wire in a suspect's car, they still didn't have a case. There was no proof that it was the telephone that had been stolen from the apartment. After all, there are millions of telephones around. The suspect stated that he had found the telephone on the street or in an alley . . . What did it matter? There was no proof to connect the suspect with the burglarized apartment. When the broken wires were examined under an ordinary microscope, they couldn't be matched to the wires in the apartment. But the scanning electron microscope revealed that the broken wires fit together perfectly, thereby linking the suspect directly to the crime.

Another crime-solving application of the scanning electron microscope is in the examination of chemicals such as paint, dye, oil, and a long list of similar substances. When a bank robber used to flee with cash, he had to be caught in the act or be definitely identified by eyewitnesses. Now, when the bank teller hands over money to a bank robber, one stack of bills may be doctored —it may contain a device, similar to a time bomb, that explodes after the bank robber leaves the bank. The explosion leaves a red dye all over the robber's clothes, car, and stolen money. This sudden experience might cause the robber to become upset and temporarily set aside his getaway plans. Alerted police can then swoop in and make an arrest. But if the robber had his wits about him, he could say that he was not the robber of the bank. If there were no eyewitnesses, the police might not have a good case. But now crime labs can test the dye on the robber and on the money and match it with the dye that was in the bank and put together a solid case against the bank robber.

Many people are familiar with the police artist who tries to convert witnesses' descriptions into a likeness of the criminal. Now there is a computerized police artist

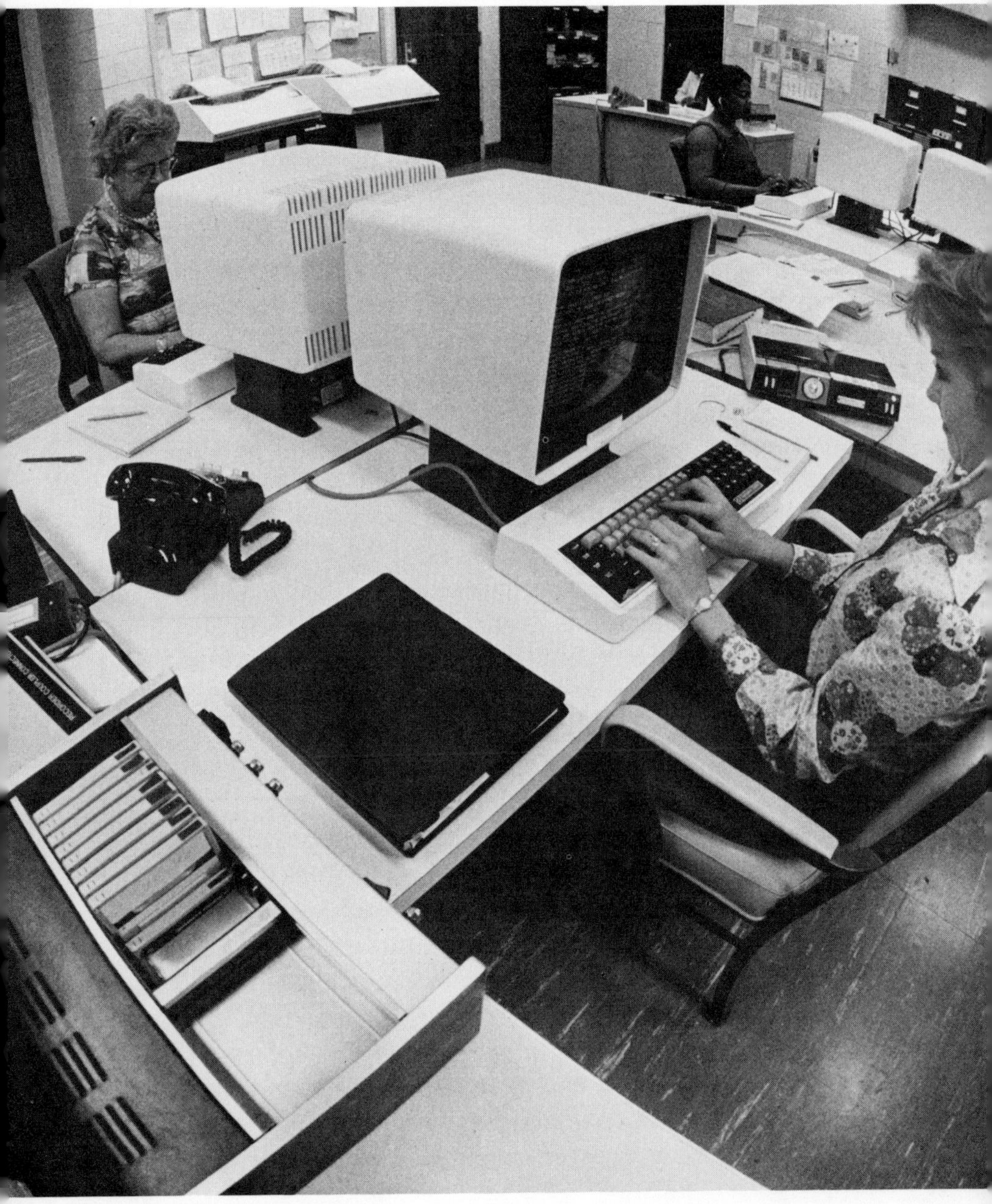

system that takes descriptions and produces a composite drawing. Then, once the drawing is made, the computer searches through police mug photographs and sorts out similar photographs. This saves hours and hours of searching by hand. When the machine is finished, the witness only has to look at photographs of people who have some resemblance to the person the witness described.

With the addition of computers to the crime lab, it now seems that the odds are beginning to stack up more and more against the criminal. Now, and increasingly in the future, the slightest piece of dust, a fallen hair, or a thread may be all that is needed to convict someone of a crime, no matter where or when it was committed.

MODERN TECHNOLOGY HAS
IMPORTANT APPLICATIONS
IN CRIMINAL INVESTIGATIONS.

BIBLIOGRAPHY

Arthur, Richard O. *The Scientific Investigator.* Springfield, Ill.: Charles C. Thomas, 1973.

Cameron, J. M., and B. G. Sims. *Forensic Dentistry.* Edinburgh and London: Churchill Livingstone, 1974.

Hall, Jay Cameron. *Inside the Crime Lab.* Englewood Cliffs, N.J.: Prentice-Hall, 1973.

Horgan, John J. *Crime Investigation.* New York: McGraw-Hill, 1974.

Kirk, Paul L. *Crime Investigation.* New York: John Wiley and Sons, 1974.

Leonard, V. A. *Criminal Investigation and Identification.* Springfield, Ill.: Charles C. Thomas, 1971.

O'Hara, Charles E. *Fundamentals of Criminal Investigation.* Springfield, Ill.: Charles C. Thomas, 1973.

Picton, Bernard. *Murder, Suicide or Accident.* New York: St. Martin's Press, 1971.

Polson, Cyril John. *The Essentials of Forensic Medicine.* Springfield, Ill.: Charles C. Thomas, 1965.

Schultz, Donald O. *Crime Scene Investigation.* Englewood Cliffs, N.J.: Prentice-Hall, 1977.

Spitz, Werner U., and Russell S. Fisher. *Medicolegal Investigation of Death.* Springfield, Ill.: Charles C. Thomas, 1973.

Walls, H. J. *Forensic Science.* New York: Praeger, 1968.

INDEX

ABOUT THE AUTHOR

A full-time writer, John F. Waters is the author of over twenty books for young people, including *Carnivorous Plants* and *Fishing* (First Books) and *Maritime Careers* (A Career Concise Guide) for Franklin Watts. A specialist in writing science books, Mr. Waters is the author of a number of books that have been named Outstanding Science Trade Books for Children by the National Science Teachers Association and the Children's Book Council. Mr. Waters, who also enjoys body-surfing and beach-walking, lives with his wife and four children in Chatham, Massachusetts.